PREPARATION FOR BREAST FEEDING

Preparation for Breast Feeding

DONNA AND RODGER EWY

DOLPHIN BOOKS
DOUBLEDAY & COMPANY, INC.
GARDEN CITY, NEW YORK

Library of Congress Cataloging in Publication Data

Ewy, Donna.
    Preparation for breast feeding.

    Bibliography
    Includes index.
    1. Breast feeding.   I. Ewy, Rodger, joint author.
II. Title.
RJ216.E86   649′.3
ISBN 0-385-08962-7

Library of Congress Catalog Card Number: 74-33606
        Copyright © 1975 by Donna and Rodger Ewy
                All Rights Reserved
        Printed in the United States of America

FOR

Marguerite, Suzanne, Rodger, and Leon

With special thanks to Roberta Scaer

Foreword

There have been many important scientific contributions to obstetrics and pediatrics in the past ten years. Yet, one of the most significant improvements in the care of newborn babies has been the rediscovery of the human breast as a source of infant nutrition. How odd that we have had to relearn nature's lesson. There is now ample evidence of the many nutritional, medical, and emotional benefits of breast feeding. Moreover, there has been a "grass roots" return to breast feeding throughout this country so that in many areas up to 75 per cent of women express an interest in nursing their newborns. To match this renewed interest by both the medical profession and prospective mothers, there now has been written this very sensible, sensitive, and knowledgeable book for the nursing mother. The case for breast feeding is presented enthusiastically but fairly, the problems of nursing dealt with soundly one by one, and the frustrations of the new mother are anticipated and provided for.

Donna and Rodger Ewy have combined a unique talent for communication and a profound understanding of the importance of the family. This together with a thoroughly researched and admirably illustrated text has resulted in this superb manual for the mother who desires to breast-feed her infant. The book will also be of great value to medical personnel who seek solid, practical aids in counseling the breast-feeding mother.

Watson A. Bowes, Jr., M.D.
Professor of
Obstetrics and Gynecology
University of Colorado
Medical Center

Preface

Like millions of new mothers and fathers before us, my husband and I were in full mutual agreement: No parents had ever created a baby as beautiful as our newborn daughter. As we looked at her we were sure that we were the first human beings to have ever had such an extraordinary experience. Her tiny fingers and toes, her perfectly shaped head, and her body were all sculptured to perfection. We were ecstatic.

As the doctor left us alone with our baby, my ecstasy gradually turned to concern. Not only had I expected to breast-feed our new baby, but I had also expected the process to be programmed into being a mother. As I put her to breast, I soon became aware that I had never seen a baby breast-feed—let alone been part of the experience myself. Unaware even that my milk wouldn't come in for three days, I somehow bumbled through the first days, hoping that things would miraculously become better.

The next few weeks were anxious ones. A multitude of problems came and went, products of ignorance—and solved by sheer desperation. Did I have enough milk? Why was my baby crying? What should I do? My lack of knowledge was overwhelming. My own mother had not breast-fed her babies, nor had any of the friends near me. I was dismayed with my inexperience and my ability to care for our newborn. Instead of enjoying the experience as I thought I would, I was besieged with feelings of inadequacy and lacked confidence in my ability to care for this baby whose life was in my hands.

My husband's love and support was constant and, fortunately, as time passed I became increasingly more proficient at breast feeding my baby and actually began to enjoy my experience as a mother. After six weeks my daughter and I were well on the road toward becoming experts at getting and giving nourishment. As I looked back at the beginning weeks I was only sorry that it took me so long to get the knowledge and confidence to enjoy the experience.

When my next three babies were born, breast feeding was a joy. I knew what was happening, what to do, and how to do it. I felt happily confident in my role as a mother and looked forward with pleasure to nursing each child. My babies sensed my confidence and reflected the joy we all felt.

PRENATAL INSTRUCTOR

Although my own children are now well past the breast-feeding stage, as an instructor of prenatal classes for more than ten years, I am still in contact with new mothers and my compassion and sympathy accompany them with the birth of their first babies. Couples who come to me radiant with the birth of their newborn fresh in their minds call me in desperation a few days later with pleas for information about feeding and caring for their babies:

"My baby has been crying all day—what should I do?"

"I don't know if I have enough milk."

"My milk isn't rich enough for my baby."

"My breasts are sore and swollen."

"How do I know if I'm feeding my baby enough?"

They are searching for help and support and they have the feelings and concerns I felt with my first baby.

Throughout my experience, I have become increasingly concerned with the number of mothers who wanted to breast-feed their babies and, because of lack of knowledge, confidence, and support, were faced with failure. It has become evident that women are expected to undergo some marvelous transformation to competent, proficient, and spontaneous motherhood, when their first baby is born. Common sense tells us that competency and proficiency come only with knowledge, confidence, and experience.

PLEA FROM THE NURSES

My own impressions of breast feeding were reinforced at a recent meeting of the Nurses of the American College of Obstetrics and Gynecology where as the authors of *Preparation for Childbirth,* my husband and I had been invited to talk about the Lamaze method of childbirth. Conversation, however, turned from childbirth to breast feeding. The nurses discussed their concern about patients who wanted to breast-feed:

"I feel as a maternal nurse that breast feeding offers a baby the best start he can get in life, however, I am concerned with the number of women who come to us after childbirth so excited with the birth of their babies and so unprepared for breast feeding."

"Although they are enthusiastic about breast feeding, they seem to be totally unprepared, both physically and mentally, for the experience."

"Of course, some women have no problems with breast feeding, but I am concerned with the number of new mothers who give up trying after they go home from the hospital."

The more we discussed our feelings, the more aware we became of the need for a well-organized, low-keyed, and realistic approach to breast feeding. As we contacted doctors throughout the Denver area, we became more enthusiastic about putting together such a manual to help new mothers.

ROBERTA AND BOB

Since the art of breast feeding is an enjoyable family experience, we felt that a clinical, textbook approach would not impart the feelings of warmth and joy we have had with our own experiences. And so we decided to follow a young couple through pregnancy, childbirth, and the first weeks at home with their new baby. We wanted not only to document the necessary knowledge about the mechanics of breast feeding, but also to make clear the necessity of the support and confidence a woman gains through her relationships with her husband, her family, and her friends.

Bob and Roberta Scaer are our good friends, and Roberta was in her fifth month of pregnancy when we asked them if they would be interested in co-operating in such a venture. Their enthusiasm was heartwarming. "Of course," Roberta said. "We have enjoyed breast feeding in our family and if we could help other new parents we would be delighted."

SEMINAR ON NEW MOTHERHOOD

Because breast feeding is emotional as well as physical, we felt the most important and supportive information would come from new mothers themselves. So we started a seminar for new mothers to come together to share their experiences, concerns, and feelings with each other. They were provided with an environment where they could gain knowledge to solve their problems, and where they could share their experiences in a group. Unpleasant situations turned into enjoyable ones, frustration turned into confidence, and feelings of failure into feelings of success. The enthusiasm that emanated from this group was exciting. Why shouldn't all new mothers get a chance to share their experiences?

Everyone we contacted imparted the same enthusiasm and willingness to share with others their knowledge and experiences—doctors, nurses, new mothers, and new fathers. Their contributions made this manual a reality. There are many excellent books on the over-all aspects of nursing. Since we are especially concerned with the mothers who have problems during the early stages of breast feeding after the birth of their babies, this book is dedicated primarily to the first weeks of establishing breast feeding.

Contents

Chapter 1—Introduction

Why Is Preparation for Breast Feeding Necessary?
Advantages of Breast Feeding

The birth of a baby is probably one of the most creative, fulfilling, and challenging experiences of your lifetime. However, birth is only a momentous occasion; parenthood is an investment of a lifetime. Many parents are not prepared for the many changes and challenges that accompany the birth of a new baby.

Being a parent is a learned role. Research has shown repeatedly that animals who are isolated from their parents never learn to be parents themselves. And daughters who are isolated from their mothers never learn the art of mothering. It has been only in the last one hundred years mothers have not handed down the art of mothering to their daughters, and fathers the art of fathering to their sons. In the large, extended families of the past, girls observed their mothers, aunts, and sisters mothering their babies, and learned naturally from them. In our society now, a new mother often has had only her own mother to observe and may barely remember her with babies.

All too often the baby that is placed in its mother's arms is the first baby that a new mother has ever held and cared for. "How do you hold a baby, change him, bathe him, and most important of all, feed him?" Feeding a new baby is one of the most important roles a mother has to assume. Many women gauge their success or failure as mothers by their ability to nourish and comfort their babies. Whether a woman decides to breast-feed or bottle-feed her baby, she finds she must have knowledge and support to carry out this vital role.

Today, many young parents who want their babies to be breast-fed become frustrated when they find that desire is not enough. They expect both babies and mothers to know instinctively how to find and provide nourishment. They find that they have entered parenthood without sufficient preparation. If there is a generation gap in our society, it is this lack of passing down the skills of motherhood—especially in the area of breast feeding.

WHY IS PREPARATION FOR BREAST FEEDING NECESSARY?

"Man is the greatest success of biological evolution to date" and breast feeding is part of the story of the "long and remarkable history of the way man acquired attributes which make him uniquely successful in life." Nature, the Great Realist, is concerned primarily with the survival of her species. Since the dawn of human life, mankind has been dependent on the fact that Nature not only provided a mother with the capability to nourish her baby with elements necessary for survival before it was born, but equipped her with the capacity to nourish her baby from birth until the child was old enough to take nourishment by himself. Imagine where we would be now if our ancestors were not able to provide this vital function.

What greater confidence can a woman have in her ability to breast-feed her own baby than the knowledge of the obvious ability and success of her ancestors. Until the last century, mankind thrived upon babies who were nourished by their mother's milk. Women were confident of their ability to nourish their babies because there was no other way. They were knowledgeable about the art of breast feeding because they had grown up seeing their mothers breast-feed their own babies. They received the support of everyone around them—their husbands, friends, mothers, grandmothers, sisters, and doctors.

Appalled at the childbirth mortality rate during the last century, the medical world became aware of the value and necessity of sterilization. New medical procedures and anesthetics were introduced to make childbirth less hazardous and more comfortable. The event of childbirth was taken from its unsterile and perilous area of the home into the antiseptic area of the hospital. Thanks to the medical profession the mortality rate of mothers and their babies was drastically cut.

Unfortunately, hospital procedures often were contrary to establishing breast feeding. For many years heavily anesthetized births were not uncommon. A sleepy baby and a sleepy mother are not very interested in breast feeding. It was not unusual to delay first nursing experiences and establish rigid four-hour feeding schedules with supplemental bottles. Women sometimes spent up to ten days in the hospital for childbirth and, after a period of this regime, were often discouraged from nursing their babies. At the same time, sterilization and refrigeration made it easy for a woman to give up breast feeding. As breast feeding is a "learned" art, it didn't take many generations for it to become a "lost" art.

We hope this manual will help close the "generation gap" for those women who wish to breast-feed their babies and are searching for information.

ADVANTAGES OF BREAST FEEDING

As a woman approaches the birth of her baby, the question of how she is going to feed her newborn looms large. Young mothers and fathers are becoming increasingly aware of the advantages of breast milk for their baby. Breast feeding is not only a physical act but also a mental one. Although almost all women have the physical equipment for breast feeding, their mental attitudes are vitally important in the final decision on whether to breast-feed. Before you choose breast feeding, you should understand its advantages and have firmly planted in your mind the reasons that helped you choose this method. You should be realistic about the task before you, and prepare for the energy, time, diligence, and perhaps discomfort that may exist during the first few weeks it takes a new mother and her baby to establish the milk supply.

Nature provides both physical and emotional rewards to a mother who has had a pleasurable experience with breast feeding. She realizes a special meaning of womanhood and feels confident within herself that she is providing the best nourishment possible for her baby.

ADVANTAGES TO THE BABY.

The advantages of breast feeding are many, but the greatest are those to the baby, who receives the most perfect food given to him in the most perfect way—close to his mother's body, cuddled in her arms.

Human Milk Is the Perfect Food for Human Babies. No one has denied the superiority of breast milk over cow's milk for a baby. Premature and sick babies thrive on it. Scientific research can get us to the moon but can only come close to reproducing mother's milk. Breast milk has well-documented advantages over cow's milk. Among the few you might consider:

Breast milk contains more vitamin C, vitamin E, thiamin, riboflavin, and vitamin D than raw cow's milk.

Cow's milk has a much higher content of phosphorus, sodium, and calories, which can precipitate serious problems with an overloading of minerals in a newborn's system.

Breast-fed Babies Have Lower Incidences of Allergies, Respiratory and Intestinal Diseases, Dental Problems, and Colic. Because cow's milk differs chemically from human's milk and because a bottle and nipple differ mechanically from the mother's breast, research shows that breast feeding protects your baby against a variety of complications which can occur from the effects of bottle feeding:

Cow's milk is very allergenic and contains antibodies against which the newborn can become highly sensitized. Breast-fed babies have a lower incidence of allergies such as infantile eczema, asthma, and hay fever.

Breast milk provides substances which prevent invasion of bacteria and virus into your baby's body, protecting him against respiratory and intestinal infections. Breast milk also gives added protection against vomiting and diarrhea.

Breast-fed babies tend to be less prone to obesity in childhood and later life. The higher caloric content of formulas causes babies to gain weight rapidly, and we now know that fat babies tend to become fat adults with accompanying susceptibility toward high blood pressure and heart diseases.

Breast-fed babies tend to have fewer dental problems later on. When nursing from a bottle, a baby is forced to thrust his tongue forward to control the flow of milk that jets forth from the soft rubber nipple. Tongue thrusting can sometimes cause a deformation of the palate and push the front teeth forward, remedied later only by expensive braces.

Period of Natural Resistance. Colostrum, the first substance the baby receives from the breast before the milk comes in, naturally flushes out the digestive system and provides him with the perfect transition from intra-uterine nourishment to mother's milk. It contains five to six times the amount of protein as later milk and has one half the carbohydrates. Colostrum gives the baby a temporary natural resistance to certain viral and bacterial infections which cause colds and diarrhea. Colostrum and breast milk provide your baby with antibody protection against polio, meningitis, and myocarditis.

Emotional Benefits. Psychologists are becoming increasingly aware of the tremendous significance of touching, fondling and cuddling, and skin contact to the emotional growth of a new baby. An interaction takes place between mother and baby that can create for the child the capacity for love in infancy and in later life. Although a mother who bottle-feeds her baby can provide the necessary closeness, breast-feeding ensures a natural way for your baby to receive these vital ingredients for his emotional development.

ADVANTAGES TO THE MOTHER.

Not only babies gain from the advantages of breast feeding, but mothers also enjoy both physical and emotional benefits as well.

Physical Benefits. A new mother may be surprised to experience the intensity of uterine contractions that take place when she begins to nurse her newborn. The hormones secreted during breast feeding stimulate the uterus to contract to its normal size more rapidly than in a nonbreast-feeding mother, diminishing uterine bleeding after childbirth and lessening the chance of hemorrhaging.

Emotional Benefits. Research is beginning to show that the secretion of the hormone prolactin, along with the accompanying holding and touching of the baby are responsible for fostering "mothering" feelings. This same hormone has a pleasant and tranquilizing effect on the mother while she is breast feeding. Some women may experience a pleasant sexual stimulation while they nurse their babies.

Night Feedings Easier. Night feedings are much more convenient. No preparation, heating, or sterilization is necessary.

Less Effort After Breast Feeding Is Established. Breast feeding takes less effort than bottle feeding. Time and energy spent sterilizing, preparing, and heating formula is eliminated. A mother who breast-feeds has a constant supply of sterile milk, of the highest quality and always readily available.

Less Concern. Concern over the exact formula is eliminated. A mother who breast-feeds knows she is giving her baby a perfectly formulated nourishment at the right temperature and consistency, sterilized by nature, available at the right time.

More Economical. When you visit the supermarket to check prices on prepared formulas, bottles, and accompanying paraphernalia, the economical aspect of breast feeding becomes obvious. Research has shown that totally breast-fed babies do not need solids until they are four to six months old.

More Pleasant Diaper Duty. Completely breast-fed babies produce a stool which is light-colored and smells somewhat like cheese. Not until formula or solids are introduced into the diet do stools take on an unpleasant odor.

Chapter 2—The Importance of Support

Be Your Own Best Supporter
Your Husband's Support
Your Family's Support
Your Friends' Support
Group Support
Support from Your Doctor
Myths of Breast Feeding

Success at breast feeding is dependent upon a woman's confidence in her ability to feed her baby. After childbirth a woman is especially vulnerable to support or criticism. Anxiety, fear, embarrassment, anger, guilt, and lack of confidence are all common emotions of a new mother, and especially of a mother who is trying to breast-feed. These emotions, unfortunately, can inhibit the hormones vital to breast feeding.

The manner in which a baby is nourished is a culturally approved phenomenon. Women who breast-fed their babies in the past were supported by their husbands, mothers, families, friends, and doctors. With all that support it would be difficult (if not embarrassing) not to have a good experience. Today, a woman who wants to breast-feed must actively search for those who will support her. Research has shown that if a woman has the support of her husband, family, friends, and doctor, she is almost always assured of a good breast-feeding experience. Surround yourself with knowledgeable people who have a positive attitude toward breast feeding. They will offer you invaluable support, confidence, and information. However, you can't live in isolation. Be prepared to answer the questions and doubts those around you may have.

BE YOUR OWN BEST SUPPORTER

Successful breast feeding is related to the commitment with which you enter motherhood. If a woman does not want to breast-feed and her husband does not want her to, there is no reason why she should even consider it. She can give her baby all the loving, cuddling, and touching the baby needs while giving him a bottle. The decision to breast-feed is not just an intellectual one; it is an emotional one as well. Many of the reservations that women have about breast feeding are based on misinformation, lack of information, and misconception. Many women do not breast-feed because they fear that their attempt may end in failure, that they will lose their figures, or that their activities will be hampered. Recognize and analyze any doubts which you may have and base your final decision on accurate information.

"I'M AFRAID OF FAILURE."

"I can't do it, and I'll be a failure as a woman if I try and don't succeed." Inability to breast-feed is caused by a combination of poor information, absence of knowledgeable help, and lack of support. To some women breast feeding is so natural that no preparation, knowledge, or support is ever needed. The chances of a successful experience are very good if a woman does get information and good support. But, whether you feed a baby by breast or bottle, you cannot fail as a woman as long as you love your baby.

"WILL I LOSE MY FIGURE?"

Whether you choose to breast- or bottle-feed, inheriting genes that predispose you to a good figure is your best guarantee of one. Next to that, diet and exercise are the most important factors in contributing to a trim figure. Research shows that if you wear a good, well-fitted bra throughout pregnancy and nursing, you sometimes come out with a better figure than you started with. Some women find that because of the extra caloric output, breast feeding has a slimming effect on their bodies. The greatest destroyer of a good figure is not pregnancy, childbirth, or breast feeding; it is lack of proper diet and exercise. Mothers who breast-feed their babies and overeat ruin their figures. Mothers who breast-feed and eat normally can keep their figures. Mothers who breast-feed and curb their intake of sugar, starches, and carbohydrates can improve their figures.

"BREAST FEEDING IS IMMODEST."

Women who breast-feed are not about to exhibit their breasts to the public. However, most of us are liberated enough that we won't be banished to the bedroom every three hours. A blouse or dress with buttons down the front or a well-placed blanket or shawl has allowed all of us to nurse when the situation has demanded. You can breast-feed and still be as modest as you wish.

"WILL MY SEX LIFE SUFFER?"

Not if you don't let it. You shouldn't let the baby stand (or sleep) between you and your husband. Make the arrival of a baby concurrent with the enhancement of your sex life. Learn about what pleases your husband and tell him what pleases you. Be honest if stitches hurt or you are still sore from childbirth. Tell him how much you care, but give yourself a little time to get over the experience of childbirth. Silence provokes growing apart and the birth of a baby can drive a wedge into a marriage rather than pull it together. Don't let this happen. Open up new avenues of communication. Talk about feelings, pleasures, and problems; don't hide them.

"WILL I BE CHAINED DOWN?"

Although some women truly enjoy a full-time job as mother, many of us balk at a job that puts us on demand around the clock. Women who have worked or who have had outside interests are especially concerned with giving up this freedom. A common complaint is "I feel pent up. I've got to get out, I've got to be me." Don't feel guilty, you aren't abnormal. When women lived with extended families, there was always a grandmother, mother, or sister to help give the new mother a breather. You *should* get out. Follow your interests and be yourself. Make up your mind now that breast-feeding won't make you a martyr.

If you plan to breast-feed and you are sincerely committed to it, you will have to spend four to six weeks establishing the delicate balance between your baby's needs and your milk supply. But once your breast supply is established, you can leave your baby with a sitter and a supplemental bottle. You are not tied down. Breast-fed babies can go to restaurants, shows, picnics, movies and concerts, travel on planes, buses, and boats with ease. Feeding is simple everywhere you go.

"CAN I WORK?"

Even working mothers are able to breast-feed. In our modern society, many mothers aware of the advantages of breast feeding want to nurse their babies, but they also want to continue their profession. Dr. Lee Salk, author of *How to Raise a Human Being* and a prominent figure in child psychology, implores mothers to wait six months before returning to work. But some mothers must return to work before then. If so, they don't have to give up breast feeding. Many mothers, once they have established their milk supply, are able to work outside the home and breast-feed too. Once a mother has her baby on a schedule, she can breast-feed right before she leaves for work in the morning (say at eight o'clock), either leave a supplement for the twelve o'clock feeding, or, if she works close to home, come home at lunchtime for the feeding, and then breast-feed her baby immediately upon her return from work at night. Admittedly, it is more difficult and more work and hassle, but it can be done.

"HOW LONG DO I HAVE TO BREAST-FEED MY BABY?"

A woman should only breast-feed her baby as long as she enjoys the experience. Because of the immunity factors a mother can pass on to her baby the first six weeks are the most vital. However, that is usually the period it takes a new mother and her baby to really become proficient. Some women nurse their babies a year or more, and others only six weeks.

YOUR HUSBAND'S SUPPORT

It can safely be said that breast feeding is a fifty-fifty proposition. A woman who is supported by her husband can almost always have a successful breast-feeding experience. A husband who encourages his wife to breast-feed is one of the greatest contributors to her confidence and ability to overcome obstacles. With the wholehearted support of her husband, a new mother can surmount tremendous obstacles; uncommitted doctors, bad hospital experience, negative family and friends. A husband who wants his wife to breast-feed can offer the best support by:

1. Understanding the mechanism of breast feeding.
2. Giving his wife full physical, mental, and emotional support.
3. Assuring his wife of his confidence in her.
4. Protecting her from people and experiences that might damage her confidence in herself.
5. Protecting her from situations that will cause exhaustion or tension.

If a husband does not approve of breast feeding, a woman should reconsider her decision to breast-feed. However, because men are as conditioned by society as women, many husbands may be negative to breast feeding because they have never thought about it and are somewhat reticent to even discuss it. Before a wife gives up her attempt, she should try to find out why her husband does not want her to breast-feed and expose him to some informative material which will help him make a more educated decision.

You are not the only one vulnerable to misconceptions and misinformation. Much of your husband's fear of, or support of, breast feeding is colored by his own experiences—or lack of them. If he comes from a family or a background that has never considered breast feeding, his conception will of course be completely different from that of a man who has come from a family that accepts it as a normal function. If your husband has negative feelings about breast feeding, they may be a product of his background, or be based on lack of information.

Find out how your husband feels about breast feeding. If he has negative or noncommittal feelings, find out why. Supply him with as much information as you can concerning the importance of his role in breast feeding. Probably the most helpful ally you can find is another man, preferably a friend of your husband's, who has enjoyed the experience in his life.

"WILL A BREAST-FEEDING BABY THREATEN OUR RELATIONSHIP?"

Probably the most common reason that a husband subconsciously fears breast feeding is that the baby will threaten the relationship between him and his wife. A wife should be aware that she must reaffirm her husband's importance in his mind. She must remind him of how important he is to her and what a unique role he fills in her life. The birth of a baby is a traumatic change, and the wife must take special pains to make her husband feel of prime and unalterable importance in her life.

"I DON'T WANT MY WIFE SHOWING HER BREASTS IN PUBLIC."

Men who come from a background where breast feeding has never been practiced may fear that breast feeding is immodest. If these feelings exist, the husband must be made to understand that complete privacy and modesty can be attained with dresses and shirts that button up the front, along with a discreetly positioned shawl or blanket. A husband who at first is extremely concerned with his wife showing her breast in public becomes more relaxed after a few weeks, with the naturalness of his baby receiving nourishment from his wife's breast.

"WILL BREAST FEEDING LIMIT OUR ACTIVITIES?"

Some men have natural concerns that breast feeding will limit their social activities. The changes that a baby can bring to a man's life are traumatic and very few men wish to change their lives completely because of a six- or seven-pound new charge. Those men whose wives have breast-fed their babies find that they can go anywhere, at any time, with built-in bottle, formula, and sterilizer. Camping, hiking, and outdoor activities are naturals for a nursing baby. It is easy to take your newborn to concerts, car races, restaurants, or movies. Just as babies and mothers differ, so do fathers. If your husband wants to get out alone with you, go out and leave a supplement. Both you and your husband will feel much better if you do. Once your supply has been established, there is no reason you can't take the day off for skiing or other activities. Nurse right before you go, leave a supplemental bottle, and nurse when you get back.

YOUR FAMILY'S SUPPORT

Your feelings about breast feeding are vastly influenced by how your own mother chose to feed her babies. If your mother breast-fed her children, you are apt to have positive feelings about breast feeding and are more likely to have a positive experience in nursing your own baby. The greatest help a mother can give her daughter is to pass down the art of breast feeding. However, if your mother did not breast-feed her children, she is more helpful if she:

1. Encourages her daughter to seek helpful information.
2. Supports her daughter's decision to breast-feed.
3. Refrains from making discouraging remarks (especially if she tried to breast-feed and failed).

If your mother did not succeed at breast feeding, she may share with you the problems she encountered. Instead of being intimidated by her experience you can be sympathetic with the reasons for her failure, and avoid them yourself.

"I DIDN'T HAVE ENOUGH MILK."

Your mother was probably a victim of the archaic hospital system in which mothers were overanesthetized for a birth and the baby was kept away from the mother for a long period of time, put on a four-hour schedule and given supplements. She is right, she didn't have enough milk—because the milk glands were not stimulated to produce the milk her baby needed for nourishment.

"MY MILK WASN'T RICH ENOUGH."

A victim of misinformation, your mother probably wasn't told that breast milk is thin and bluish in color. Mother's milk is consistent in the quality, nutrients, minerals, and vitamins a baby needs. It is the mother who suffers from a deficiency in her diet. A mother's milk is much easier for a baby to digest than a cow's milk and therefore satisfies the baby's appetite for a shorter period of time, causing a breast-fed baby to be fed at more frequent intervals.

"I WAS TOO NERVOUS."

Most mothers tend to be nervous about caring for a newborn, and nervous tension inhibits the let-down response. Had your mother understood how important the let-down reflex was, she could have taken steps to encourage relaxation and a positive attitude before each feeding.

"MY BREASTS WERE TOO SMALL."

(And you are shaped just like your mother!) Breast size has nothing to do with successful breast feeding. Unromantic as it appears, large breasts are a result of fat tissue, not milk glands. Women who are liable to have the most difficulty are those with large, pendulous breasts.

YOUR FRIENDS' SUPPORT

Your peer group has a great influence on you from the ages of five to ninety. No one is more sympathetic and helpful to a new mother in her attempts to breast-feed than a friend who has breast-fed her own babies and is able to offer advice, encouragement, and support. For the first few weeks, surround yourself with friends who support breast feeding and especially those who have successfully breast-fed their babies and can give you help, positive advice and support when you need it. Don't give up your other friends, but do try to circumvent the subject of breast feeding with those who are negative or uninformed about it. Nothing can be more deflating than some friend who can, with one innocent comment, cut down your confidence in breast feeding.

"IT WAS TOO PAINFUL."

Women can undergo excruciating pain because of lack of preparation and knowledge, and by letting preventable problems get out of hand. Many doctors feel that if a woman prepares her breasts before the birth of her baby she can forego cracked and sore nipples. The pain of engorgement and infected breasts after birth can be alleviated by knowledge of prevention, drainage, and proper treatment.

"MY MILK DIDN'T AGREE WITH MY BABY."

Medical research shows that mother's milk is carefully formulated to suit the baby's needs. A premature or sick baby actually thrives on breast milk. Milk banks have been called on to help these babies survive. Babies with allergies in their families are better off with breast milk. However, a mother who is extremely nervous, harassed, and lacking in confidence in her ability to supply enough milk for her baby may be vastly relieved to turn to a prepared formula because then she knows exactly what her baby is getting and how much.

"MY BABY WAS PREMATURE."

Premature babies may not have the mouth muscles developed enough to be able to suck as well as a full-term baby. However, through hand expression (or a breast pump) a diligent mother can provide breast milk for her baby until he can suck well enough on his own. Doctors are especially concerned with the weight gain of premature babies. If the weight loss is significant and it is a matter of survival to your baby, some doctors recommend that the mother continue nursing and supplement the premature baby's diet until he is strong enough to suck well, although it is evident that this is twice as much work for the mother.

"MY BABY WAS BORN BY CAESAREAN SECTION."

Caesarean section means a general anesthetic, a sleepy mother, and a sleepy baby. However, once the mother and baby have recovered from the effects of anesthesia they both can apply themselves with as much fervor as after an unanesthetized birth.

"YOU HAVE TO WATCH WHAT YOU EAT."

Usually breast-feeding mothers can eat anything they want to, including chocolate, spices, tomatoes, or onions—and the baby is no more concerned than when he was in your uterus and you were eating these things. However, once in a while a mother may find that after she has eaten onions or garlic, for instance, her nursing baby may be restless. Or after she has eaten chocolate or candy, her baby may have diarrhea. She simply leaves these foods out of her diet for a few weeks until her baby's system develops enough to handle them. Even substances as potent as nicotine and alcohol must be consumed in prodigious quantities to get through to a baby.

"THE BABY WILL BITE YOU."

Most babies begin teething around four to six months. If and when a baby does get his teeth and accidentally bites down, your involuntary sharp "No" quickly stops him. He wants to nurse, and he won't persist in doing something that produces a negative reaction in his mother.

"I CAN'T STAND THE THOUGHT OF A BABY HANGING TO MY BREAST EVERY MOMENT."

New mothers do have a tendency to overnurse their babies. Out of ignorance, frustration, and desperation they set up a common pattern that would drive a saint wild. On a two-hour schedule, they allow the baby to nurse on one side for one hour and then switch him to the other breast and allow him to stay on the other breast for an hour. Then they look up at the clock and realize it's time to start over again. The baby approaches this next feeding with a nonchalant attitude and diminished appetite and starts the whole cycle over again. From the time you put your baby to breast, it takes about three minutes to stimulate the let-down reflex, and seven more minutes for your baby to get almost all of the milk out of each breast. Throw in another five to ten minutes at each breast to satisfy his sucking needs. About fifteen to twenty minutes on each side is plenty of time to nurse a baby. The experienced mother then burps her baby, puts on a dry diaper, makes sure he is comfortable and then allows him to digest what he has in his system. A baby accepts a mother who is sure of herself and definite in her intentions.

GROUP SUPPORT

In the past, new mothers had support from their mothers, sisters, and grandmothers. Women in our society who breast-feed their babies often feel that they are alone in their endeavors. They don't know where to turn during moments of frustration.

Many new mothers find it extremely helpful to be able to get together with other mothers who are willing to share their experiences. In many communities helpful groups may be contacted through your local hospitals, health centers, Red Cross, YWCA, and La Leche League.

Several years ago a group of women who were convinced of the advantages of breast feeding joined together to help other women who wanted to breast-feed their babies. They called themselves the La Leche League. This group has given much encouragement and support to many mothers who were ready to give up breast feeding because of lack of information, lack of confidence, and lack of someone to turn to for help. League leaders are available twenty-four hours a day for counseling and can provide medically approved information on anything from engorgement, sore nipples, and supplements to nursing twins.

SUPPORT FROM YOUR DOCTOR

A doctor who is a sympathetic and active supporter of breast feeding is one of the important factors in helping a woman to have a positive breast-feeding experience. He is the person the woman turns to for knowledge, support, and confidence. When a doctor tells a woman he is confident of her ability to breast-feed her child, he bolsters her confidence 300 per cent. A supportive doctor gives a new mother knowledge about her ability to produce milk, about the importance of let-down, and about the significance of drainage. Before the birth of your baby choose your obstetrician and pediatrician or family doctor carefully. Find out how they feel about breast feeding. If you have an obstetrician have him recommend a pediatrician or family doctor who would be sympathetic with your views.

Today, many doctors are convinced of the advantages of breast feeding. They know that they must advise, counsel, and support if their patients are to succeed in the art of breast feeding. Although it may take more of a doctor's time and effort at first, he is well rewarded by appreciative mothers and fathers and by society, as a supporter of a generation of women and men who are confident and happy with their roles as parents.

MYTHS OF BREAST FEEDING

Myths about feeding have caused many women to be defensive about their choice. Many women are frightened to begin breast feeding because of misinformation and misconceptions.

"IF YOU DON'T BREAST-FEED, YOU HAVE FAILED AS A MOTHER."

Whether breast feeding or bottle feeding, a mother who loves her baby can only *succeed*. Love covers the multitude of mistakes we all make as new mothers. *With love there can be no failure in motherhood.*

Many women choose to bottle-feed their babies because in our society they feel uncomfortable with the concept of using their breasts.

Some women do not breast-feed because their husbands do not want them to. Some women cannot breast-feed successfully because they do not have sufficient confidence, knowledge, or support. And, for one reason or another, a small minority of women simply aren't able to provide enough nourishment to sustain their babies. The love, touching, closeness, and fondling that are so vital to a baby's emotional growth and that naturally accompany breast feeding can also be provided by the mother who bottle-feeds her baby and is knowledgeable about the importance of these elements.

"ALL WOMEN SHOULD BREAST-FEED THEIR BABIES."

The success of breast feeding is directly related to the commitment on the part of the mother. A woman who chooses to breast-feed her baby should do so because she really desires to and thinks she will enjoy the experience. Because breast feeding is an emotional as well as a physical experience the choice to breast-feed should definitely be up to only the mother and father. If a woman does not want to breast-feed her baby, she should not be pushed into a role at which she will surely fail.

"ALL MOTHERS CAN BREAST-FEED EQUALLY WELL."

It is only realistic to realize that some women will produce more milk than others. A few women just seem to be "naturals" at it. They effortlessly produce copious amounts of milk. But most women become proficient at breast feeding only after they have gotten some helpful knowledge and support. Others have to work prodigiously at it. No mother should feel guilty about breast feeding! It is not an endurance game, nor is it a platform for martyrdom.

"ALL BABIES NATURALLY KNOW HOW TO BREAST-FEED."

Babies differ in their ability to nurse. A mother may be surprised that she had plenty of milk for her first baby, but doesn't have such a good experience with her second one. The mother who assumes all the responsibility for getting nourishment to her baby may feel guilty about what she assumes is her own lack of ability, when in reality it is her baby who has not learned to co-operate in the feeding process. It takes two to tango and just as some mothers are proficient nursers, so are some babies. Some babies need to be taught the art of breast feeding and it may require a great deal of patience.

"BREAST FEEDING IS EASIER THAN BOTTLE FEEDING . . ."

Many a new parent has been led down the path of ignorance with this unfinished statement, only to be discouraged by the reality of the left-out part *only after breast feeding has been established.* Establishing the breast-feeding pattern between mother and baby may take more knowledge, energy, and patience than bottle feeding. However, mothers who do establish the pattern not only enjoy the experience, but also reap the rewards of a built-in milk supply best suited to their babies' needs.

"BREAST FEEDING IS A NATURAL METHOD OF CONTRACEPTION."

The belief that breast feeding provides a safe interval of contraception is not too well received by those of us who have conceived while breast-feeding. However, if a baby is totally breast-fed (that is, no supplements, water, solids, or even pacifiers are given), breast feeding causes hormones to be secreted which tend to suppress ovulation (the release of an egg for fertilization) for about seventy-five days postpartum, and it postpones the resumption of the menstrual cycle for seven to fifteen months. The consensus is "Don't count on breast feeding for contraception; talk to your doctor for the best kind of contraception for you."

Chapter 3—Knowledge

Milk Production
Let-Down
Milk Drainage
Demand and Supply

With an understanding of the mechanics of breast feeding, a woman and her husband have the basic knowledge and techniques to cope with the realities of breast feeding.

Without knowledge young mothers fall victim to problems that would discourage the most stalwart soul, problems that could have been alleviated and minimized in the first place, problems that, with immediate care, can be cleared up quickly, and problems that, without treatment, can lead to failure at breast feeding.

Milk Production. An understanding of how her body is equipped to produce milk gives a woman an appreciation of and confidence in her ability to nourish her baby without concern.

Let-down. One of the most important basics of breast feeding is an understanding of how a woman's system works to get the milk from the breast to the baby. Because the process of let-down is dependent upon a balance between her nervous system and hormonal system, a woman must protect herself from the many factors that can threaten this delicate balance.

Proper Drainage. The most serious of the problems that lead to ultimate failure in nursing is an ignorance of the importance of establishing and maintaining proper milk drainage. With an understanding of this process, a mother is able to avoid possible pitfalls.

Proper Care of the Nipples. Many women experience such discomfort with their nipples that they cannot continue their breast-feeding endeavors. With knowledge, a woman is able to prepare herself before

Milk Production

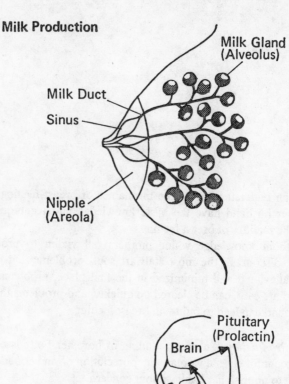

Milk Gland
(Alveolus)

Milk Duct

Sinus

Nipple
(Areola)

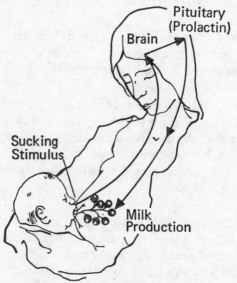

Pituitary
(Prolactin)

Brain

Sucking
Stimulus

Milk
Production

FIG. 1 MILK PRODUCTION

the birth of her baby, prevent problems before they occur with the first nursing experience, and treat the problem if it does occur.

Training of the Baby. Breast feeding depends not only on a willing mother, but also on a willing and able baby. Many simple techniques of handling an unwilling or unable baby can avert a potentially unpleasant situation.

Complications and Problems. There are possible complications and problems that may arise in any breast-feeding situation with a new baby. A realistic and knowledgeable approach help both a woman and her husband to cope with the problems, and know where to turn for help.

MILK PRODUCTION

The remarkable production of milk from the nutrients of your blood into milk perfectly suited to your baby's needs is made possible by the glands which produce the hormones necessary for this miraculous transition.

Breast milk is made by clusters of ten to twenty glands which are called alveoli (al-ve-o-lee). These glands are located deep in the fatty parts of the breast. During pregnancy, when large amounts of progesterone and estrogen are present in your bloodstream, these milk glands grow larger in expectation of their role of producing milk after your baby is born. After birth, the sharp decrease of the hormones signal the milk glands to begin their task—that of producing milk for your baby.

However, there are two participants in this production of milk—you and your baby. The presence of milk glands themselves is not enough. When your baby begins to suck at the nipple, the sensitive nerve endings in the nipple send a message through your nervous system to your brain, which stimulates the pituitary gland, the master controller of emotions. The pituitary secretes a hormone called prolactin, which is then secreted into your bloodstream. It is this hormone (sometimes called the mothering hormone) that reaches the milk glands and signals them to begin their production of milk. The glands begin to make milk a few seconds after the baby begins to nurse. However, this milk remains in the milk glands, still out of the reach of the baby, ready for

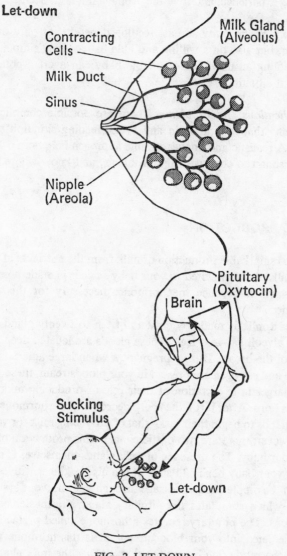

Let-down

Contracting Cells

Milk Duct

Sinus

Milk Gland (Alveolus)

Nipple (Areola)

Pituitary (Oxytocin)

Brain

Sucking Stimulus

Let-down

FIG. 2 LET-DOWN

the next step in the miraculous production of milk. The milk must then be let-down, or squeezed, from the milk glands, through the milk ducts and finally into the milk sinus (or reservoir), where your baby can get to it.

The first substance to come from your milk glands is *colostrum*. Colostrum is a somewhat thick, sticky, yellowish material that comprises the first nourishment your new baby receives. Its most important function is to transfer to your baby immunities you have developed over your lifetime. It has a slightly laxative effect that helps your baby's system rid itself of the residues formed in his previous home, the uterus. There is some indication that colostrum also acts as a protective agent against diarrhea. Because your baby is born with an excess of fluids in his system, it is normal for him to lose a few ounces during the first few transitional days after birth.

Your true milk will come in about two to four days later. It takes from seven to fourteen days to really establish milk production. And it sometimes takes about six weeks for a new mother to refine her techniques and begin to feel some expertise in breast feeding.

The true milk looks rather thin and bluish and is sweet-tasting. It contains all of the vitamins, minerals, and nutrients your baby needs to survive. The milk seems to be of constant quality regardless of the mother's health. Nature provides that the baby gets all the nutritional elements he needs from his mother's body. There is evidence that although your baby may not suffer seriously from a poor diet, you will. A nutritionally sound diet puts back into your body what you have used to produce milk.

The significance in your understanding *milk production* is that you may be confident that you were born with the capability of producing milk of the quality and quantity your baby needs to survive. The size of your breasts has nothing to do with your capability to produce milk.

LET-DOWN

Remember that making milk is not only a physical process, but also an emotional one. Though almost all women have the physical equipment to make milk, the emotional aspect is what makes breast feeding an enjoyable experience or a frustrating one.

The problems a woman may encounter come somewhere between

making the milk and getting it through the milk ducts and into the sinus where your baby can get to it. This process is called the let-down.

Around each *milk gland* are bands of muscular cells (called myoe-phithelial cells), which are responsible for squeezing the milk out of the glands through the milk ducts and into the sinus. About two to three minutes after prolactin has caused the milk to be produced, the continuing sucking stimulus of your baby at the nipple is sent through the nervous system to the brain, where it signals the pituitary gland to once more send out another hormone called *oxytocin*. Oxytocin is a hormone that causes muscular cells to contract; it is the same hormone that caused the muscles of your uterus to contract during the birth of your baby. This hormone is sent through the bloodstream, and in a few seconds it reaches the milk glands, where it causes the muscular cells around the glands to contract and squeeze the milk out of the glands.

The milk is passed through the *milk ducts* and into the *milk reservoir* (usually called the *milk sinuses*), which are located under the dark area of your nipple (the areola). Here it is easily available to the baby.

This is a beautiful, if rather delicate, system of balance of your nervous system (the stimulus sent to the brain) and your endocrine system (the prolactin and oxytocin sent through the blood stream to the milk glands).

However, there is one snag in the process. Because the let-down is an integral part of the brain process, it is affected by other emotions as well. If you are tense, fearful, anxious, angry, or embarrassed (all common emotions for a new mother), your pituitary sends out other hormones which can inhibit the effect of the oxytocin. There you are, with your breasts full of milk and a hungry baby who can only par-tially get to it. Even though the milk glands are capable of producing copious amounts of milk, without the let-down reflex, your baby can't get sufficient milk to meet his needs, resulting in an unsatisfied, hungry, crying baby and a frustrated, nervous mother. And, of course, the more upset a mother is, the less she is able to experience the let-down function. A vicious cycle can be set up which may end in an unsuccessful nursing experience.

The let-down is a reflex function. Once breast feeding is established, a mother may find that the cries of her baby at feeding time are enough to cause the let-down. It is usually preceded by a tingling sensation or a pins-and-needles feeling in the breast. Some women say they feel a sudden fullness in their breasts when they experience the let-down. A sure sign of let-down is when the milk actually begins streaming from the breast. This streaming or leaking lasts only until the muscular walls of the breast become elastic enough to handle the surplus milk. Leaking can be controlled by placing firm pressure, with your hand or your forearm, against the breast. As your milk does not come in for several days, do not be concerned if it takes some time for the let-down reflex to begin functioning smoothly.

Although almost every woman is capable of producing milk without conscious effort, the let-down function is in your control. If you want an enjoyable experience, take special care to ensure that you approach each nursing session with a calm, relaxed, and positive attitude. Before you begin to nurse your baby, take time to set up a pleasant situation. Reserve this time for yourself and your baby. Pamper yourself. You are a very special person doing a very special thing.

Because our society puts considerable pressure on new mothers, this let-down function is probably one of the most sensitive of the breast-feeding mechanisms. A woman's ability for let-down may be impaired by the inherent rush, bustle, and hustle of everyday life, combined with lack of knowledge and an unnatural attitude about women's breasts.

MILK DRAINAGE

The milk ducts have the all-important job of transporting the milk from the glands into the sinus. If drainage is maintained, they function without problem. However, they signal distress immediately if, for some reason, their mission has been interfered with.

EARLY (TISSUE) ENGORGEMENT.

When your milk supply comes in, some two to three days after birth, the milk ducts are called upon to carry milk from the glands to your baby. The ducts accomplish this mission easily if the walls that surround them are elastic enough to allow the passage of milk. (Swelling and hardening of breast tissue is caused by milk being released into inelastic ducts.) If the walls of these vessels are too rigid they

Maintain Drainage

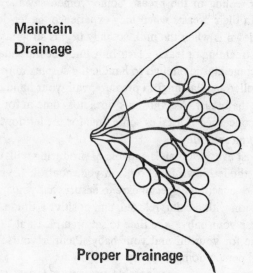

Proper Drainage

Obstructed
Milk Duct

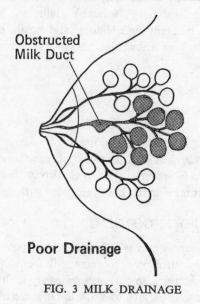

Poor Drainage

FIG. 3 MILK DRAINAGE

obstruct the passage of milk. When the milk comes in with force, the milk ducts simply are not stretched enough to cope with the amount of fluid. The breasts become swollen and tender when the extra fluids from your blood and lymphatic system come rushing to the area. Blood and lymph pumped into the tissue cause increased tension, which blocks even further the milk ducts. This early engorgement condition usually develops about the third or fifth day after a baby is born, and lasts about forty-eight hours. Many doctors feel this situation can be prevented by a combination of massaging the breasts and hand-expressing the colostrum to condition the milk ducts during your pregnancy and putting the baby to breast as soon as possible after birth. Ultimately, the milk ducts will become stretched and have a greater capacity for handling the milk load. At the same time your milk supply will become balanced with the demands of your baby. When this engorgement passes, the swelling of the breast tissue subsides and many women are concerned that they have "lost their milk." It only signifies that the ducts have developed the capacity to cope with the milk supply.

MILK ENGORGEMENT.

It is essential, however, to maintain drainage throughout your breast-feeding experience. Later engorgement may take place at any time if anything interferes with adequate drainage. A woman may experience such engorgement if her baby nurses only infrequently, for short periods, and cannot adequately drain the milk ducts, or if she uses supplements to the extent that the baby is not able to empty her breasts.

MASTITIS.

Just as with milk left out of a refrigerator, if the milk is allowed to stagnate in the glands it may produce infection in the breasts (mastitis). Sometimes, if your baby only partially empties the milk glands, leaving one duct unemptied, a small, red, streaked lump in your breast may signify that just one duct has become plugged and susceptible to the complications that may occur with engorgement. This type of engorgement, brought on by infrequent and inadequate drainage can be prevented by nursing on a frequent schedule and making sure the breast is emptied at each feeding.

Demand and Supply

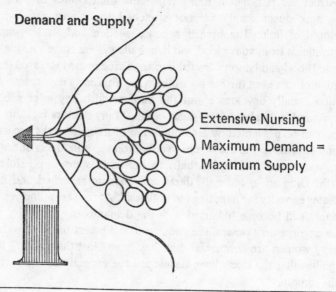

Extensive Nursing

Maximum Demand =
Maximum Supply

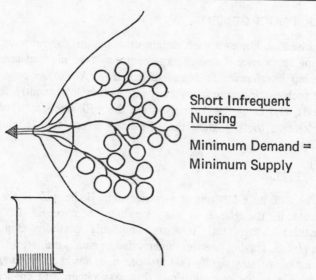

Short Infrequent
Nursing

Minimum Demand =
Minimum Supply

FIG. 4 DEMAND AND SUPPLY

DEMAND AND SUPPLY

The greatest concern most new mothers have is, "Will I be able to produce enough milk for my baby?"

How much milk are the milk glands capable of producing? The milk glands of an average woman have the capacity to produce an almost infinite amount of milk. A healthy mother can produce more milk than her baby needs. However, the production of milk is dependent not only upon the mother, but also upon her baby. The amount of milk produced is determined by how much milk is sucked out. Remember that your milk glands are stimulated to produce only when your baby sucks at the nipple. They continue producing only as long as he continues nursing. The more he nurses, the more the glands are able to produce. This is the reason women can nurse twins, and, in other cultures, women are able to nurse not only their own babies, but others' babies as well.

Women who have twins set up a schedule which fits them best. Some women nurse both babies at the same time, cradling one baby in each arm and letting their legs overlap. Other mothers may prefer to breast-feed one twin at each feeding while bottle-feeding the other.

Nature provides a perfectly balanced system: When your baby needs food he naturally increases your production ability. The more your baby nurses and empties the breasts the more your milk glands are stimulated to produce milk.

Many new mothers, unsure of their capability to breast-feed, try to give their babies a bottle to be sure they are getting enough nourishment. The more the baby's demands are met by a supplement the less sucking stimulation there is to produce milk. Mothers who use solids too early find that they dull the baby's appetite and, of course, the less demand, the less supply. Solids given before four months are beneficial only to the food manufacturers.

An experienced mother knows that the few extra hours she spends in developing her milk supply in the first few weeks will be well worth the extra time she gains in the following months. Once the milk supply is established you are able to miss a feeding and use supplements without detrimental effects.

Chapter 4—Preparation

Nipple Preparation
Nipple Conditioning
Breast Massage
Hand Expression
Inverted Nipples

Not all women have to prepare their breasts for nursing. Some women, especially those with dark hair and complexion, seem to be able to nurse their babies with no preparation and no problems. Others of us, especially redheads, blondes, and fair-skinned women find that preparation helps to alleviate sore nipples and engorged breasts. Studies show that women who prepare their breasts and nipples before the birth of their babies have a much higher success rate, fewer complications, and greater confidence than those who don't. Also, a woman who learns how to prepare her breasts becomes more familiar with handling them, and is more able to cope with problems which may arise later.

NIPPLE PREPARATION

One of the most common problems a woman may encounter with her first nursing experience is sore nipples. Some tenderness is quite normal at first and will pass within the first few days. However, preparation can help prevent the problem from getting out of hand. Women in primitive cultures seem to have few problems with sore nipples. In our society because breasts have been covered and protected, it is natural that the nipple area can be tender. Starting to prepare your nipples before the baby is born helps desensitize them. Some doctors claim that mothers who do these exercises faithfully will not have sore and cracked nipples.

Begin preparation six to eight weeks before the birth of your baby. The first essential is a good, well-fitted nursing bra even before the baby is born. Drop the flaps on the nursing bra to allow the nipple to rub against the cloth of your shirt a few minutes each day. At the same time to condition the nipples expose them to direct sunshine for a few minutes each day. During you daily bath or shower, rub your nipples with a rough terry cloth. Do not use soap, harsh cleansers, or alcohol as they have a tendency to dry out your nipples and can magnify future problems.

NIPPLE CONDITIONING

Grasp your nipple between your thumb and forefinger and gently but firmly pull until you feel a slight discomfort, then gently roll the nipple between your fingers. Repeat several times (see fig. 16). Apply lanolin, hydrous lanolin, or AandD ointment to help your nipples become more supple during pregnancy.

BREAST MASSAGE

Because we know how important it is to keep the milk ducts drained, breast massage is a good technique to help establish the flow of colostrum and drainage of the ducts. Breast massage and hand expression help to make the ducts less likely to plug up, to make the milk ducts more elastic for drainage, and to establish the flow of colostrum. Starting at the base of your chest where the breast is fullest, place a hand on each side of your breast, with thumbs and fingers of both hands together (see figs. 17 and 18). Then gently but firmly slide your hands together toward the nipple. Repeat this several times. You are now ready to continue with the technique of hand expression, which will help you throughout your nursing experience.

HAND EXPRESSION

Holding your left breast, grasp the nipple with you right hand (see fig. 19). Place your thumb on top and your forefinger under the dark area of the nipple that surrounds and covers the milk sinus. Then gently push your finger and thumb back toward your chest (see fig. 20), and without sliding them toward the nipple, compress them together to squeeze out any fluid which you massaged down to the sinus under the nipple (see fig. 21). Move your finger and thumb clockwise a quarter of the way around and squeeze again. Grasp your right breast with right hand and with your left hand continue to squeeze at points corresponding to the twelve- , three- , six- , and nine-o'clock points on a clock. If you do not emit a drop of colostrum with your first attempts, keep trying and eventually you will. If you have special difficulty, ask your doctor or nurse to show you how to do it.

It should be mentioned here that because some doctors believe there is only a "limited" amount of colostrum available, which should not be "wasted" by hand expression before the birth of a baby, you should check with your doctor on this practice. After the birth, however, you will find hand expression most helpful in the case of engorgement and for supplements.

INVERTED NIPPLES

Most women's nipples naturally become erect when the baby begins to nurse, so he can grasp the nipple easily. Some women, however, have nipples that tend to remain flat and even a little inverted—that is, they sink into the breast. When a nipple does not become erect, it is difficult for your baby to grasp efficiently for nursing. Your doctor can tell you if your nipples have a tendency to be inverted or you can determine it by examining yourself: Grasp the nipple between your thumb and forefinger (as in the nipple conditioning) and gently pull out. Usually the nipple will remain erect; however, because nipple inversion is caused by adhesions, an inverted nipple will tend to shrink in rather than to stand out. Completely inverted nipples are rare; however, if you have a tendency to inversion, start a regime of working with your nipples about eight weeks before your due date. The nipple pull and roll are very good to break the adhesions which are holding your nipples in. Besides the daily firming exercises you can wear a plastic shield inside your bra to help the nipple stand out (see fig. 22). The Woolrich shield has two parts: the base, with an opening for the nipple, is fitted against the breast and exerts a pressure which eventually holds the nipple out; the top covers the nipple, but stands away from it. Women with inverted nipples who have worn these shields feel that they do help.

Chapter 5—Beginning Breast Feeding

Childbirth

The First Nursing Experience

Establish Early Realistic Breast-Feeding Expectations

Emotional Changes in the Hospital—First Three Days

CHILDBIRTH

Successful breast feeding begins with the birth of your baby. Research has shown that the baby should be nursed as soon as possible after birth. In a normal, uncomplicated birth, both baby and mother benefit from early nursing. After birth, the newborn is experiencing his first impressions of the outside world. Early nursing provides him the warmth of his mother's body, the touch and feel of her skin, the sound of her voice and heartbeat, the continuation of a nourishing substance, and his first accomplishment outside the uterus of sucking at her breast. If he is put to breast within the first hour of his life, a baby usually has the instinctive reflex to suck. If he is not, this reflex diminishes and does not return until forty hours later. If there are complications, such as a heavily sedated or Caesarean birth (after which the mother and baby are both sleepy) or a premature birth (after which the baby is too weak to suck, and keeping him warm is of utmost concern), the baby's first nursing experience is left to the discretion of the doctor.

There is evidence that the first hour after childbirth is critical not just to the baby but to the mother as well. Holding the baby and marveling at her creation seems to provide a woman with emotions that have profound effects on her feelings about her baby and about herself as a mother (see fig. 23). Many mothers who have had their babies taken away from them at birth experience feelings of depression and rejection.

A baby born of a primitive mother instinctively grasps for the warmth of its mother's body and for her breast, and the mother instinctively nestles the baby to her breast, not only for psychological reasons, but for physical as well. One of the dangers of the period right after the baby is born is hemorrhaging from where the placenta has detached itself from the walls of the uterus. When the baby starts to suck at the nipple, the stimulation causes the hormone oxytocin to be released into the mother's bloodstream. This chemical, which causes the muscular cells of the milk glands to contract, also causes the muscles of the uterus to contract to shut off the open areas left from detachment of the placenta. So early nursing actually helps the uterus of the mother to return to its normal size more quickly and reduces the chances of hemorrhaging.

The father also benefits from this period of closeness between the mother and baby. The man who can touch, feel, and handle his newborn is much more likely to accept the reality of his role as a father.

THE FIRST NURSING EXPERIENCE

Although a baby naturally searches for his mother's nipple and a mother naturally reaches for her young, many things can happen between the searching and the reaching that can enhance the breast-feeding experience.

EMOTIONAL PREPARATION.

First and foremost, try to approach breast feeding in a relaxed and positive mood. Look to your doctor, nurse, and husband for support in helping you attain a positive attitude and protect you from the negative feelings that might strip you of the necessary confidence you need. Think of all the reasons you have chosen to breast-feed.

POSITION.

Don't start to breast-feed your baby until you are in a comfortable position. Your first nursing experience will probably be on the delivery table or in bed. Breast feeding while lying down appears to make it easier for the baby to nurse and is also more comfortable if you have stitches during delivery. Turn on your side and prop pillows under your head, shoulders, back, or wherever it is comfortable. Most women prefer to put their lower arm above their heads. Place your baby on his side beside you with his feet touching your body and his head slightly away from your breast. If you are sitting in bed, prop a pillow behind your back and under each arm and cradle your baby in the crook of your arm with his head close to your breast and his feet in your lap.

TECHNIQUE.

Leave his hands uncovered so he can enjoy the touch and feeling so important to him. Gently bring him up to touch your breast. Don't thrust your breast into his face or he will feel as if he is being suffocated and will fight to get away from the nipple (see fig. 24).

All newborn mammals are born with a "rooting reflex," which is nature's way of ensuring them survival. Whenever anything touches a newborn's cheek, he will instinctively turn in that direction and try to put the object in his mouth.

Grasp the dark area of your nipple between your thumb and forefinger and gently stroke back and forth on your baby's cheek with the nipple. Because he was born with this "rooting reflex" he will turn to grasp the nipple. Be sure he doesn't latch on only to the end but that he has the area of the nipple that covers the milk sinus. When he grasps on, slide your finger to the base of his chin and press firmly to keep the nipple against the roof of his mouth to help elicit the sucking reflex.

If your baby is nursing properly he has grasped the nipple between his tongue and the roof of his mouth, gently compressed his gums around the milk sinuses and squeezed the milk into his mouth (see fig. 25). As a slow, rythmical, satisfied sound comes from your baby, you can be confident he is nursing properly. If you have especially full breasts, you may have to press a finger against your breast by your baby's nose to leave room for him to breathe more freely (see fig. 26). When your let-down reflex is working, it is normal to feel a tingling, full feeling in your breasts and perhaps a slight tenderness in the nipples. As your baby begins to nurse, the slight tenderness disappears and you can sit back and enjoy the experience. The prolactin hormone has a tranquilizing effect and, if your baby is nursing properly, the rhythmic motion and sound is enjoyable.

DIFFICULTIES.

Some babies are "natural born" nursers, others need some coaching. If he is not a super nurser from the start, be patient with him. You may have to stroke his cheek with your nipple several times to get him to take the nipple. You may have to put the nipple in his mouth several times to get him to grasp the nipple correctly.

If a baby is allowed to nurse as soon as possible after delivery, many difficulties can be avoided. Healthy babies, whose mothers have had little or no anesthetics, usually have no problems of sucking immediately after birth. The second feeding is spontaneous for the mother and baby and they both settle into a successful pattern.

One of the most common problems a new mother may encounter is the sleepy baby who resists all efforts to wake him up. The mother is willing to nourish her baby—but the baby is not willing to nurse. Later he may awake angry and hungry but in the meantime his mother may feel inadequate and unsure of herself. A sleepy newborn may be the direct result of anesthetics which were given the mother during her labor. If this is so the mother should be assured that it is not her fault and she need only wait until the anesthetics wear off.

If your baby is just a sleepy baby, special care should be taken to bring the baby in to feed as often as possible, so his sucking will stimulate your milk supply. Before you begin to breast-feed wake up your baby. Loosen his blankets, sit him on the bed, cupping his chin in one hand, with your other hand supporting his back (just as you would when you burp him in the sitting position). Gently bend him at the waist and give him a few seconds to wake up. When he awakes put him to your breast right away.

A second common problem the mother may encounter with her newborn is the baby who is brought in screaming and when put to his mother's breast begins to scream louder. This doesn't take long to make a mother feel rejected and inadequate.

Your baby not only will not eat while he is screaming, he cannot eat, and if you stuff the breast into his mouth, he will be terrified of suffocation. Your first objective with a crying baby is not to feed him, but to calm him down. Talk to him, soothe him, caress him, rock him back and forth until he settles down, and then put him to your breast.

COLOSTRUM—FIRST NOURISHMENT.

During your first few days in the hospital, milk production is your least concern, because the nourishment your baby is receiving from your breasts is colostrum. Colostrum is the yellow, sticky substance, rich in protein, which your breasts have been producing during the last part of your pregnancy. Milk usually appears twenty-four to forty-eight hours later. However, the earlier and more vigorous the sucking stimulus the faster the milk "comes in."

THE LET-DOWN.

About three minutes after your baby is put to breast, you may feel the sudden full and tingling feeling of the let-down sensation in your breasts. During the first few days your nervous system and hormonal system may have to learn how to work together, so don't be alarmed if it takes some time. Because of the hospital situation many women don't experience the let-down until they are in the familiar and comfortable settings of their own home.

HOW LONG TO NURSE.

If you have tenderness the first few days of nursing, allow for the firming of your nipples by nursing your baby on a gradually increasing schedule. At each feeding, nurses usually suggest three to five minutes at each breast, five to six minutes the second day, and seven to ten minutes the third day, gradually increasing the time until you are nursing fifteen to twenty minutes on each side.

HOW TO TAKE YOUR BABY FROM THE BREAST.

Don't pull your baby from the breast while he is sucking. When he is nursing he sucks in your nipple between his tongue and the top of his mouth creating a tremendous vacuum which, if you pull him away while he is still sucking, can be very painful. To break suction painlessly, gently place your little finger into the corner of his mouth between the nipple and his lips (see fig. 27). If this does not naturally break the suction, push your finger in further between his gums where he is compressing the nipple.

BURPING.

During feeding, a baby can get an air bubble in his system which can cause him discomfort and make it difficult to nurse properly. The most common way of burping is to hold your baby up to your shoulder and gently pat his back until you get the desired effect—sometimes just a murmur and sometimes a surprisingly loud "burp." Holding the baby on your lap, supporting his back and head with one hand and gently rubbing his stomach with your free hand is an especially effective method of burping (see figs. 28 and 29). Try these techniques before feeding if your baby is crying, or, if he is a vigorous nurser, between feedings and after feeding. After the air bubble comes up, or adequate time passes (like five minutes) to ensure that there is no air bubble, switch the baby to the other breast and continue nursing.

CHANGING BREASTS.

Feeding at both breasts during a nursing session accomplishes two important things: It ensures complete drainage of the breasts, and it stimulates the second breast. It is important that you begin the next feeding with the breast your baby used last at the previous feeding. Use both breasts at each feeding. The baby tends to empty the first breast most completely and the second breast is usually left only partially emptied. It ensures complete drainage of the milk ducts and sinus. Since these ducts have not been employed before, they may not have the elasticity necessary to cope with the passage of colostrum and can cause engorgement.

SCHEDULES.

Remember that the first few days are transitional ones for both you and your baby. Your baby has never known schedules, and to try to force one abruptly on him now would be unwise. His little system, far from being set on a four-hour schedule, will probably call more often for some nourishment. It is not unusual for a new baby to want to eat every two or three hours, night and day. On the other hand, it is not unusual for a new baby to be fatigued and sleepy and not too interested in your breast. The most important efforts in these first few days are to condition your nipples for when your milk comes in and to try to condition and train the let-down process. Most doctors now suggest that a mother nurse her baby on demand during the first few days. This usually means nursing every two to three hours. As your baby's system matures, he usually extends this period to four hours on his own, with perhaps a little encouragement from his mother.

HOW DO YOU KNOW IF YOUR BABY IS GETTING ENOUGH MILK?

Because a baby is born with an excess fluid reserve, it is normal for your newborn to lose weight (10 per cent of the birth weight) the first few days of life. He will regain that weight if he is fed eight times in a twenty-four-hour period. When your milk comes in, you can be confident that your baby is getting enough milk if:

He Maintains a Steady Weight Gain. If you have a good-size baby who nurses well and is showing a steady weight gain you have no need to worry. The nourishment you are providing your baby is adequate for his needs. Usually small and premature babies give more reason for close attention as they do not have the same strength and muscle power to get milk from their mothers.

He Produces Six to Eight Wet Diapers a Day. What goes in must come out and since you cannot measure what goes in, you must gauge your confidence on what comes out. If your baby produces six to eight good wet diapers a day, you are pretty well assured that he is getting plenty of milk.

He Is Contented. A happy baby is the best measure and mainstay to your confidence. If a normal-size baby appears to be happy with his supply he probably is being well nourished.

The breast is capable of producing all the milk the baby needs. The amount varies in each breast from three to ten ounces, depending on the baby's demand. The baby gets most of his milk in the first five minutes and empties the breast in ten minutes.

ESTABLISH EARLY REALISTIC BREAST-FEEDING EXPECTATIONS

It takes time for both the mother and baby to establish a good breast-feeding relationship. Don't expect to be able to nurse your baby effectively right away. Many times new babies are just too sleepy to be very hungry during the first few days of life. Some babies have to be taught to grasp the nipple and nurse properly. If your hospital stay is short, your milk may not come in before you leave. Your milk supply may come in two to four days after birth and the mature milk supply is not established until five to seven days after birth.

BOWEL MOVEMENTS.

How many young mothers are prepared for their babies' complex little digestive factory? But what goes in must come out. And what comes out tells us a lot about what's going on in that little factory. The baby's first bowel movement is called meconium. It is a dark, sticky substance that looks like tar. Meconium is the intra-uterine substance that is cleared from your baby's body. After your true milk comes in, the baby's bowel movements will become light and look and smell somewhat like cheese. Normal bowel movements are runny. Babies are as various in their types of bowel movements as they are in their types of personalities. Feel confident that breast-fed babies almost never have diarrhea or constipation. However, some babies have a movement with every feeding and some only every few days. As long as the movement is moist and soft and the baby doesn't have to strain too hard, you need not worry about it.

When you start adding supplements, and especially solids, the bowel movements become increasingly darker and take on an unpleasant odor.

EMOTIONAL CHANGES IN THE HOSPITAL—FIRST THREE DAYS

Childbirth is one of the most emotional experiences of life and it is normal for both the mother and father to undergo great emotional change and stress.

MOTHER.

It is not uncommon for the mother to feel extremely elated, creative, and fulfilled. Many women are so excited that they can't sleep for hours after the birth of their baby. Under these feelings of elation, other emotions are running high. The mother may experience intermittent feelings of overwhelming responsibility, fear, and frustration that she can't cope with. She may feel insecure about being away from her husband. Some women have real feelings of discomfort with the stitches and soreness from childbirth.

THE BLUES.

Your baby is beautiful, your husband is wonderful, the nurses and doctors have been great! And you burst into tears for "no reason." The postnatal blues have hit again, unpredictable and indiscriminate. They may come two days after the birth of your baby—or two weeks. You may get them with your first baby or not until your third. Although many theories have been suggested, no one really knows what causes the postnatal blues. But considering the tremendous changes that take place in your hormonal balance after the birth of the baby, this kind of reaction isn't really surprising.

Women cope with the blues differently from using home remedies to obtaining psychological support. Your greatest help in combating the blues is to realize that they are not abnormal and they will pass. Of primary importance is an understanding husband, one who tells you he loves you and encourages you to hold on until the blues are gone. By the way, some new fathers seem to go through the blues just as mothers do, so you may have to comfort your husband. Overwork, overextension, and unrealistic expectations of yourself can bring on depression for *anyone*. Try to relax, to enjoy your baby, and to do only what work is necessary.

FATHER.

After his baby is born a new father may have feelings of joy and pride and love that may overwhelm him. However, after the baby's birth, his wife is whisked away from him, the baby is off to a nursery, and for many men it is the first time in their married lives that they have been left alone. The birth of a man's child usually leaves him fatigued; he has forgotten to eat, and no one cares.

The responsibility settles on his shoulders. The bill for the birth of this baby is just the beginning of the responsibility he must meet for many years to come. Although many women now contribute to the finances of the family, it is the father at this time who is concerned with the financial responsibility. What will his life be like now? How will his relationship with his wife change? The few days his wife is in the hospital may leave him alone, frustrated, and uneasy. Not wanting to be misinterpreted, he finds it hard to express his feelings and may remain silent and forgotten.

Chapter 6—At Home

Physical and Emotional Developments
Feeding Your Baby

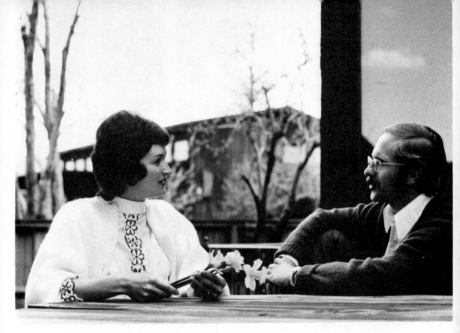

Fig. 1 ROBERTA AND BOB
Roberta and Bob discuss the significance of breast feeding the new
baby who will soon come into their family. A woman who is supported by her husband can almost always have a successful breast-
feeding experience.

Fig. 2 ROBERTA AND DOCTOR
A supportive doctor is important in the decision to breast-feed. On
an early visit, Roberta discusses breast feeding with her doctor.

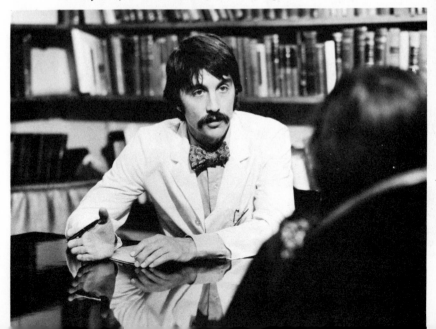

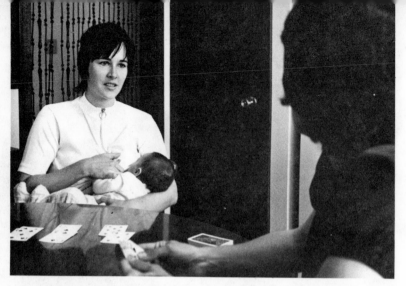

Fig. 3 ROBERTA AND SUE

One of the greatest helps to a new mother is a friend or relative who has successfully breast-fed her own child. Roberta knows she can call her friend Sue any time she runs into trouble.

Fig. 4 ROBERTA PREPARING HER BREASTS

In her seventh month of pregnancy, Roberta begins to prepare her breasts for breast feeding.

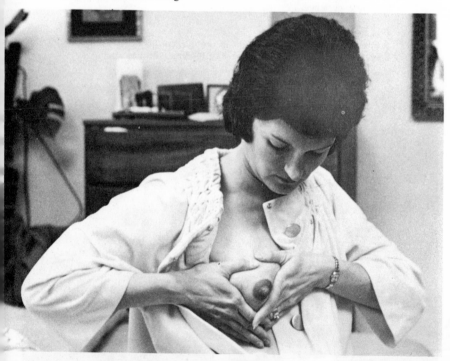

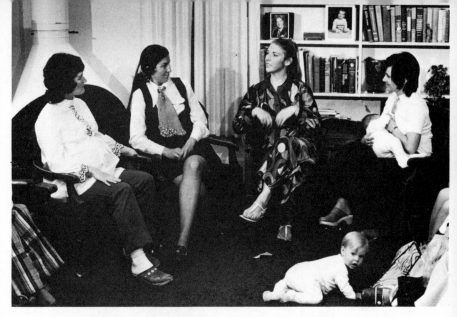

Fig. 5 ROBERTA AND LA LECHE
Searching for information, Roberta turns to a group of La Leche
mothers to give her support, confidence, and knowledge.

Fig. 6 ROBERTA IN LABOR
Bob encourages Roberta during her labor.

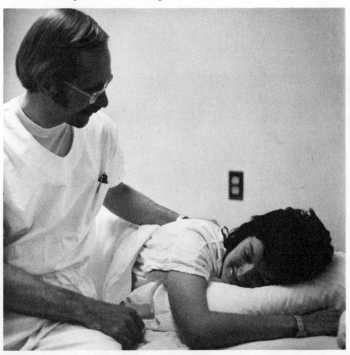

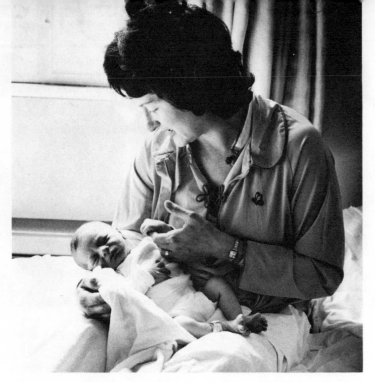

Fig. 7 ROBERTA AND ANDREW
Andrew is joyously welcomed into the world by a proud mother.

Fig. 8 FIRST NURSING
Roberta nurses Andrew as soon after birth as possible. Bob looks on
with pleasure.

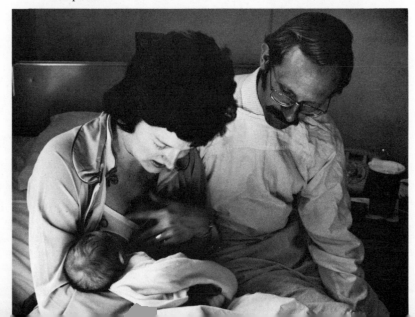

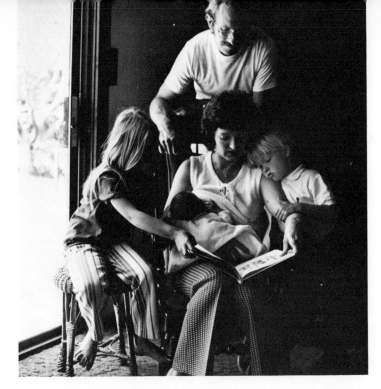

Fig. 9 ROBERTA AND FAMILY—AT HOME
At home, Andrew is soon part of the family. Roberta reads to the family while Andrew nurses contentedly.

Fig. 10 ANDREW AND MICHAEL
Nothing is more artificial to a baby than a quiet, sterile nursery. Andrew loves to be part of the normal noise and activity of the family.

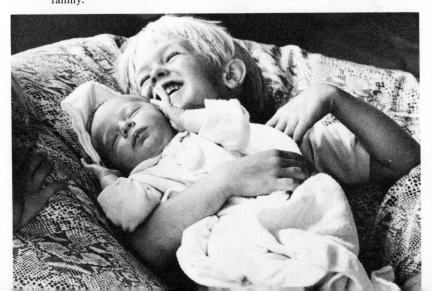

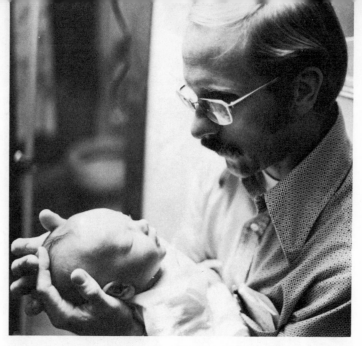

Fig. 11 BOB AND ANDREW
Bob tenderly cradles Andrew in his arms. The success of a father-baby relationship is extremely important and cannot begin too early.

Fig. 12 ROBERTA NURSING ANDREW
Roberta is confident that Andrew is receiving the most perfect nourishment possible.

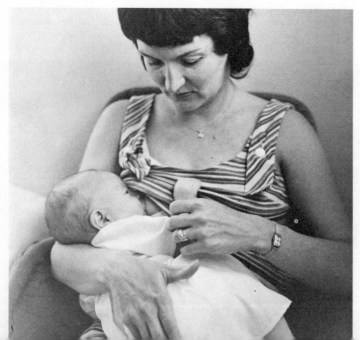

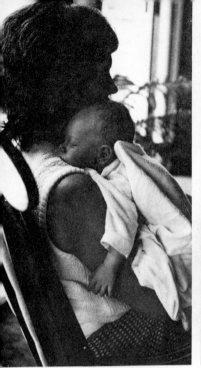
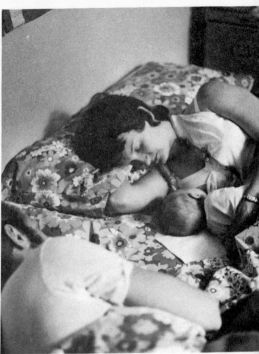

Fig. 13 ROBERTA ROCKING ANDREW
Rocking, loving, and cuddling are Andrew's first lessons of love and trust.

Fig. 14 NIGHT FEEDING
Disturbing neither his mother nor his father, Andrew enjoys the night feeding which is important to both him and his mother.

Fig. 15 A FAMILY PICNIC
A breast-fed baby can go anywhere at any time with his own built-in food supply. The family enjoys a picnic while Andrew enjoys his own dinner.

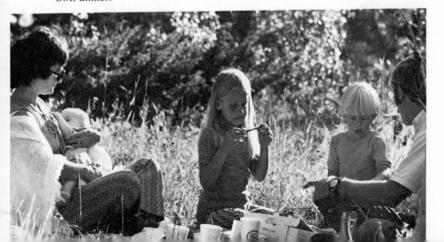

Fig. 16 NIPPLE CONDITIONING

Grasp your nipple between your thumb and forefinger and gently but firmly pull until you feel a slight discomfort, then gently roll the nipple between your fingers. Repeat several times.

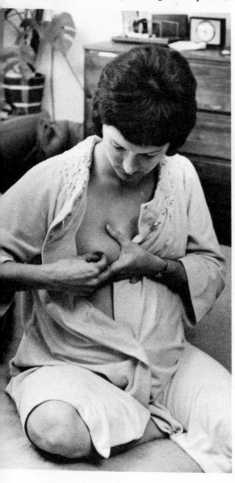

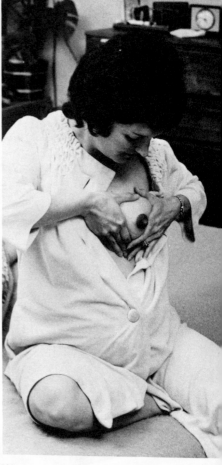

Fig. 17 BREAST MASSAGE (1)

Start at the base of your chest where your breast is fullest. Place a hand on each side of your breast, with thumbs and fingers of both hands together.

Fig. 19 HAND EXPRESSION (1)
Holding your left breast, grasp the nipple with your right hand, placing your thumb on top and forefinger under the dark area of the nipple.

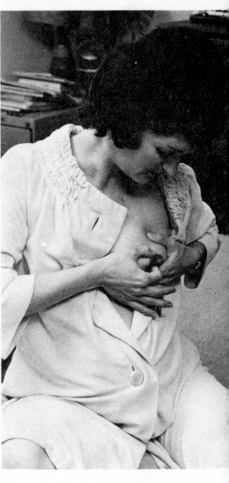

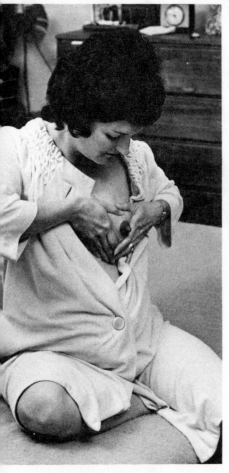

Fig. 18 BREAST MASSAGE (2)
Gently, but firmly, slide hands together toward the nipple.

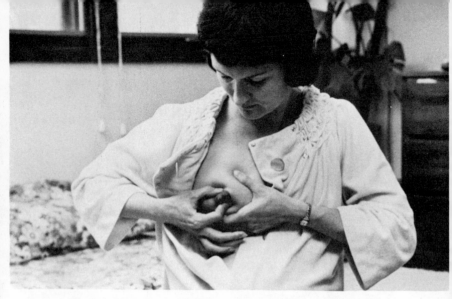

Fig. 20 HAND EXPRESSION (2)
Then gently, push your finger and thumb back toward your chest (without letting your fingers slip forward).

Fig. 21 HAND EXPRESSION (3)
Compress your fingers together to squeeze out any fluid that you have massaged down to the sinus under the nipple.

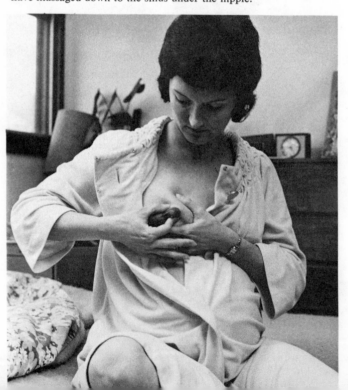

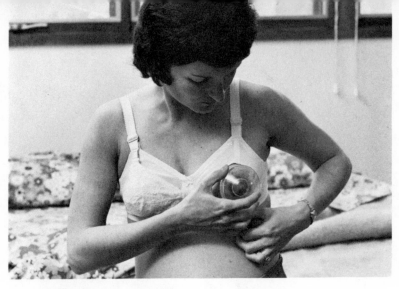

Fig. 22 INVERTED NIPPLES SHIELD
Because Roberta has a tendency toward inverted nipples, she inserts
a shield under her bra, which will help train her nipples to stand out.

Fig. 23 ROBERTA AND ANDREW
Holding and handling your baby as soon as possible after birth
seems to have profound effects on both you and your baby.

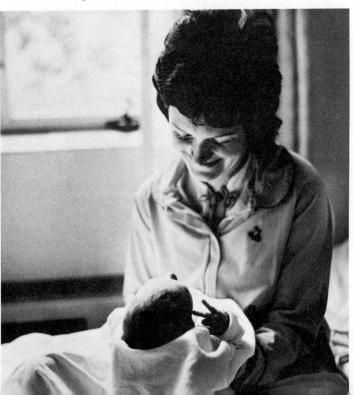

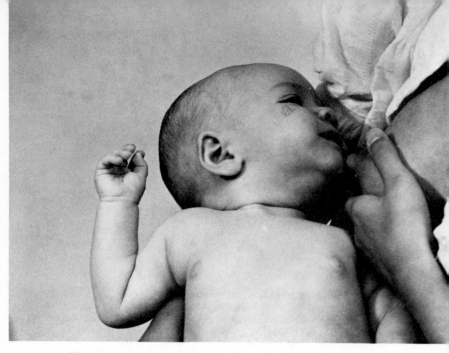

Fig. 24 TECHNIQUE
Gently bring your baby to the breast. Grasp your nipple between
your thumb and forefinger and gently stroke the baby's cheek with
the nipple.

Fig. 25 BABY NURSING PROPERLY
The baby has grasped the full nipple between his tongue and the
roof of his mouth and is nursing contentedly.

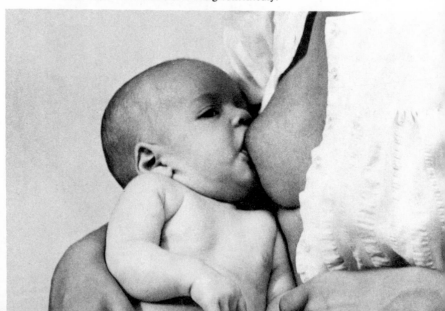

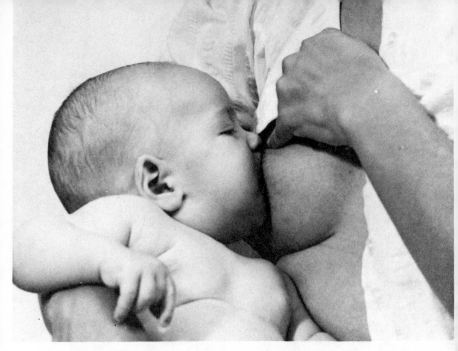

Fig. 26 FULL BREASTS
If you have especially full breasts, you may have to press a finger against your breast to leave room for him to breathe more freely.

Fig. 27 HOW TO TAKE YOUR BABY FROM THE BREAST
Don't pull your baby from the breast while he is sucking. Gently place your little finger into the corner of his mouth between the nipple and his lips.

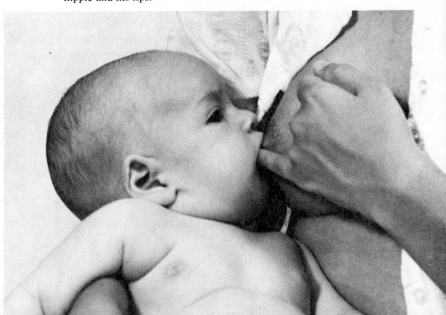

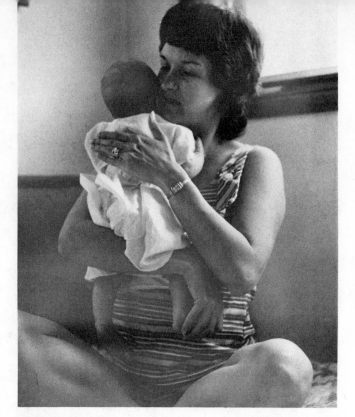

Fig. 28 BURPING (1)
Hold your baby up to your shoulder and gently pat his back.

Fig. 29 BURPING (2)
Hold the baby in your lap, supporting his back and head with one hand, and gently pat his back or rub his stomach.

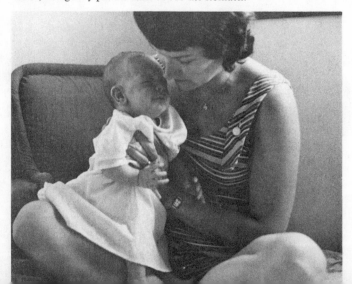

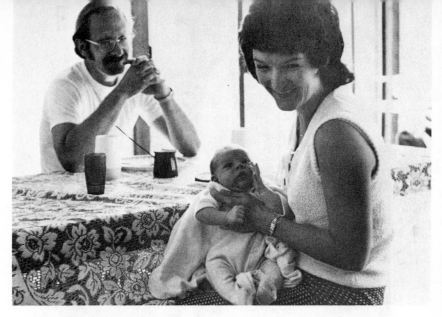

Fig. 30 AT HOME—BOB, ROBERTA, AND ANDREW
During the first six weeks of life, something goes on between baby, mother, and father that can never be duplicated.

Fig. 31 THE FIRST LESSONS OF LOVE
We know that the first weeks of life are of utmost importance in the emotional development of a baby. The first lessons of love are a natural outcome of breast feeding.

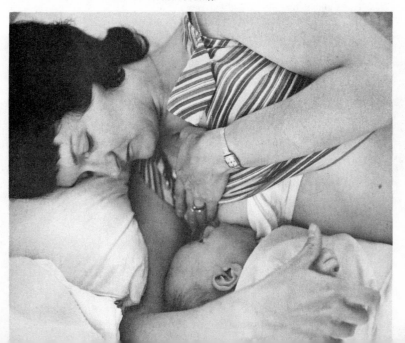

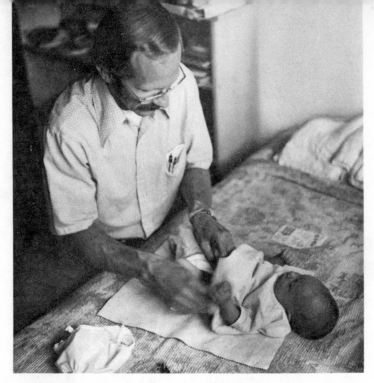

Fig. 32 BOB AND ANDREW
Your husband is your most important supporter. Encourage him to
be a part of the experience during these first few weeks.

Fig. 33 RELAXED ROBERTA AND ANDREW LYING
Relax and enjoy breast-feeding your baby.

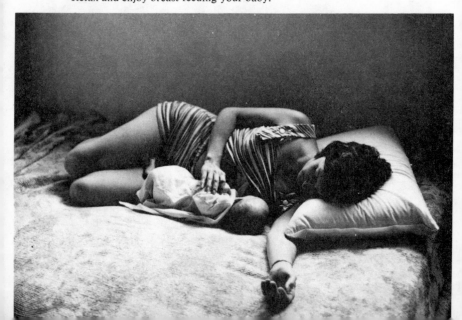

During the first six weeks of life, something goes on between baby, mother, and father that can never be duplicated (see fig. 30). Your baby undergoes not only great physical growth, but also emotional and psychological development. Your life changes overnight. Your role now incorporates that of individual person, wife, and mother. Your husband undergoes great emotional changes as well, and your marriage now includes a third being. A family who recognizes the significance of this period sets a blueprint for a lifetime.

PHYSICAL AND EMOTIONAL DEVELOPMENTS

The changes in a newborn's life are marked not by days, but by seconds at first, then by minutes. Your baby will never undergo such rapid development again in his life. His growth, both physical and emotional, during the first few weeks of life is phenomenal.

The significance of this early period of your baby's life cannot be overemphasized. He has spent nine months protected and nourished by your body. At birth he is suddenly thrust into a world of constantly changing temperatures, noises, and sensations. Remember that your baby had a very special life in your uterus. He never knew the pangs of hunger because he received constant nourishment. He never knew silence because he was constantly in touch with the sounds of your heartbeat, digestive system, and when you spoke, your voice. He knew constant motion, because when you moved he moved and when you walked he was rocked by the motions of your body. Think of the first six weeks of his life as a transitional period for your baby. Mothers who try to duplicate this life in the uterus find both themselves and their babies less frustrated. Their expectations of a new baby are more realistic, and their babies are much easier to care for. Feed him when he is hungry. Talk to him, sing to him. Hold him close to your body so he can touch you and hear your heartbeat. Cuddle, fondle, and rock him.

Your baby has one basic need—that of survival. To survive he must be provided with nourishment, protection, and love. Before birth your baby never experienced hunger, so his inability to cope with a four-hour schedule is easily understood.

We know that the first few weeks of life are of utmost importance in the emotional development of a baby (see fig. 31). Babies who don't get the stimulation of cuddling, touching, and rocking are likely to be handicapped in their later ability to love and trust. A mother and father who give their baby attention and stimulation are actually giving him his first lesson in the art of loving and being loved. If his needs of hunger and discomfort are met with love, tenderness, gentleness, and pleasure, coming always from you, he learns to form his first important attachment. The feel of your skin, the sound of your voice, and the closeness of your body are vital nutrients that ensure your baby's capacity for love and intimacy in later life. Breast feeding provides these necessary elements naturally. When a baby is being breast-fed, he is fondled, caressed, rocked, and cuddled close to his mother's body. At the same time he is receiving warm, sweet, nourishing milk. Although a mother who bottle-feeds her baby can certainly provide these experiences for him, these first lessons of love are a natural outcome of breast feeding. Needless to say, a baby who is constantly fed with a bottle propped on a pillow is being deprived of one of the most important experiences of life. Realize how important these first weeks are. Look forward to each feeding as a major experience for your baby.

FEEDING YOUR BABY

When you leave the hospital to go home, you may have doubts about your ability to cope without the help of your doctors and nurses.

Remember, first, that women have built-in capacities to nourish, care for, and love their young. Second, your husband is your most important supporter (see fig. 32). Encourage him to be a part of the experience during these first few weeks.

The knowledge you obtained before the birth of your baby and the experience you have gained in the hospital have given you a firm basis for coping with and enjoying your newborn. You will use the same techniques you learned in the hospital to nurse your baby. However, you will have the security and warmth of your own home, where your baby and you can work out your own special relationship. Your main goal these first few weeks is to establish your milk supply. If you rest, relax, and feed your baby when he is hungry you can almost always be assured of a good experience.

Most new mothers are not prepared to cope with the normal needs of a new baby. The most unrealistic expectations center around the feeding patterns of the newborn.

FEEDING SCHEDULES.

Almost all new mothers are constantly trying to push their newborn babies into waiting longer and longer periods between feedings long before the babies' systems are mature enough to handle enough nourishment to sustain them for this period. An experienced mother doesn't even look at the clock. She knows that if she feeds her newborn when he is hungry, he will naturally increase her milk supply and soon will begin to stretch out intervals between feedings.

HOW LONG TO FEED THE BABY.

Nothing is more dreary to watch than a haggard and tired new mother with her baby constantly at her breast. The inexperienced mother allows the baby to nurse for one hour on one side and one hour on the other side—and is on a two-hour schedule. The mother gets discouraged, the father disgusted, and the baby confused. A baby usually gets most of the milk the first five to ten minutes of nursing, and he can empty a breast in ten minutes. After that, he is only nursing for the slow trickle of milk which the breast is producing. Babies do have a definite need for sucking, and some babies need more than others. However, twenty to thirty minutes on each side is ample time for filling both his nourishment and sucking needs. If a mother does want to nurse her baby for longer than forty minutes her baby should be able to go longer between feeding intervals.

NIGHT FEEDINGS.

Unrealistic expectations about night feedings have left more than one new mother in tears, uncertain of her mothering ability. "When will he sleep through the night?" "I hate night feedings, I'm resentful of the baby, and I resent my husband for lying there and doing nothing." Considering your baby's intra-uterine life helps you to realize how unrealistic it is to expect him to sleep for six to eight hours without nourishment during the first few weeks. Make night feedings your special time to read, listen to the radio, or think.

Trying to fit your baby into the adult world of schedules is apt to make your baby colicky and cranky, to make you frustrated and guilty, and to upset and irritate your husband. Throw away the book; your baby should be on his own feeding schedule and it may be every two, three, or four hours. Every few weeks your baby may have a growth spurt. An older baby's digestive system can take in greater amounts of milk and therefore can last longer between feedings.

Relax and enjoy your newborn's individual pattern these first few weeks (see fig. 33). Nurse him where and when he wants it. Remember the law of demand and supply. The more you nurse your baby, the more confident you can be of your milk supply.

LEAVING YOUR BABY.

Flexibility and creativity on the part of the mother are of prime importance during the crucial period of establishing breast feeding.

During the early stages of breast feeding, the mother has to be with her baby almost as much as the baby has to be with her. A skipped feeding may not only cause painfully swollen breasts—but, milk left in the milk ducts may become a source of infection. A new mother can alleviate this by hand-expressing milk into a sterile receptacle and refrigerating it for a spare bottle, which can be used later.

Be aware that if there are allergies in your family you may want to leave breast milk rather than formula milk. Consider leaving your baby for short, frequent times between feedings rather than long, infrequent times.

GIVING A SUPPLEMENTAL BOTTLE.

Some babies take to a supplemental bottle with no problem at all. Others need a little coaxing because sucking from a bottle is a completely different technique than sucking from the breast.

If you want your baby to learn to suck from a bottle given by his father or baby sitter, don't wait too long before you introduce this experience to him.

Your baby is a "creature of habit." Coach the person who is going to give the bottle to think of the bottle as a breast. Hold the baby in a cuddling position. Make him warm and secure and introduce the bottle from the position the breast would be given. Rock, coo, and talk to the baby to make him feel as secure as if he were in his mother's arms. If it doesn't work the first time, don't despair.

WEANING YOUR BABY.

Although you usually are not thinking of weaning your baby during the first six weeks, the question will come up sooner or later. Techniques of weaning vary widely. However you should approach it in the way that is most comfortable to both you and your baby.

There are two deciding factors to weaning: First, your baby. No matter how desperately the mother wants to continue breast-feeding, at five to six months, some babies simply lose interest in their mother's breast and gradually become able to get all the liquids they need from a cup. Other infants may want to breast-feed indefinitely.

This brings in the other deciding fact—the mother who is involved both physically and emotionally. We usually suggest a mother continue breast-feeding as long as she enjoys it—be it ten weeks, ten months, or two years. However, when you decide, remember the weaning can be traumatic to both of you and it is wisely accepted that it should be accomplished in a slow, gradual manner.

If your baby is less than two years old, wean him onto a bottle so you are sure his sucking needs are satisfied. If he has not taken a bottle, give him a few weeks to become used to it.

Pick the feeding time in which your baby is least interested and substitute a bottle each day. After a week, substitute a bottle for the next lightest feeding. In a few days you may then substitute a bottle in the same manner, and complete weaning can be accomplished in a month or so. This approach not only accommodates your baby's needs, but allows your breast to stop producing milk in a gradual, natural process.

Chapter 7—Prevention

No Let-Down—No Milk
Supply Follows Demand
Maintain Drainage
Avoid Sore Nipples

NO LET-DOWN—NO MILK

The milk glands can supply copious amounts of milk, which your baby can get to only partially if the milk is not let-down into the milk sinus. Rest, relaxation, and positive attitude are essential elements to successful breast feeding. The let-down can be inhibited by fear, anxiety, and tension. So relax and enjoy nursing. The let-down function is a reflex which is within your control. You know that negative emotions can inhibit the let-down. Nursing your baby with confidence and pleasure is the greatest aid to let-down. If you are having difficulty with let-down, it is helpful to apply heat to your breasts by taking a warm shower or bath, or using a hot cloth or water bottle. Massage your breasts right before breast feeding to enhance the let-down. Let-down occurs about three minutes after sucking begins, so leave your baby at each breast for at least five minutes to establish this reflex. Frequent and flexible schedules enhance let-down in a new mother.

Some of the signs of a well-functioning let-down reflex are:

1. A slight tingling sensation as breasts are filling.
2. A feeling of tension in the breasts as the milk is let down from the glands to the ducts.
3. Milk dripping or even spurting from both nipples as the baby begins to nurse.
4. A slight feeling of tenderness from the milk pressure in the nipple which goes away as your baby begins to nurse and equalize the pressure.
5. A sensation of uterine contractions as your baby is nursing is full proof that the same oxytocin, which is causing the uterus

to contract, is also causing the muscular cells around the milk ducts to contract.

SUPPLY FOLLOWS DEMAND

The less demand, the less supply. The more demand, the more supply. Milk can only be produced when the baby sucks at the nipple and the breasts are emptied. The more your baby nurses, the more milk will be available to him. If you are concerned that you do not have enough milk for your baby, your best insurance is to put him to breast more frequently to stimulate more milk production. Babies have a growth spurt around six weeks. At this time, he simply needs more milk, and the only way to develop a more plentiful supply to satisfy his appetite is more frequent and prolonged feedings. There is usually a period of forty-eight hours between your baby's increased demand and your milk supply replenishment.

MAINTAIN DRAINAGE

Milk flow, or drainage, not milk production, is necessary for successful breast feeding. When the ducts leading from the milk glands to the sinus become blocked by not being drained, they tend to become engorged and, if left uncared for, can become infected. Early, frequent nursing is the best formula to keep your breasts from becoming engorged. Nurse at both breasts as soon as possible following birth. Nursing at each breast every two to three hours helps establish drainage of colostrum and maintain milk yield. Some doctors feel that mastitis (infected breasts) can be prevented; first, by prevention of sore or cracked nipples where the infection may enter; second, by establishing good drainage so a milk duct cannot become clogged; and third, by not letting yourself become so tired and dragged down that you are open to infection. Put your baby to breast frequently to clear the clogged duct. Early and frequent nursing the first few days before the true milk comes in has several beneficial effects:

1. It helps to establish the let-down reflex.
2. It tends to make the ducts leading from the milk glands to

the sinus more elastic and less conducive to causing breast engorgement.

3. It helps your baby to become more proficient in nursing before the true milk comes in.

AVOID SORE NIPPLES

In our society, which tends to hide and cover the nipple area, the first experiences with breast feeding may lead to painful nipples. Although not every woman has a problem with sore nipples in pregnancy, women with light hair and fair skin tend to have this problem. The clue to avoiding it seems to lie in the area of prevention. Instead of going through excruciating pain that defeats the strongest desire to breast-feed, a woman should be aware of the steps to take to keep her nipples from getting sore.

The first sign of healthy nipples is that they are firm enough to stand the first nursings of your newborn. The nipples do not crack or bleed from nursing. And, although a bit of tenderness is normal, it usually goes away when your baby begins to nurse.

Preparation during pregnancy can condition your nipples. A regime of manipulating the nipples, begun some eight weeks before the birth of your baby, can help them withstand the baby's sucking. Never use soap, alcohol, or any strong substance on your nipples before or after birth, as it tends to dry them out and encourage cracking. During pregnancy use Massé, hydrous lanolin, or AandD cream to help make the nipples more supple.

Nurse frequently for short periods at the beginning to allow for toughening of the nipples. Use your common sense about the time you allow your baby to stay at the breast. If you have sore nipples, leave your baby at the breast only three to five minutes on each side the first day and increase it by several minutes each (five to six the second; seven to ten the third, and ten to fifteen by the fourth day). By that time your milk probably will have come in and you have desensitized your nipples and yet have nursed long enough to establish the let-down reflex. If you let your baby start nursing on the less sore side to stimulate let-down, then switch to the sore side so the baby can get the most out of it in the least amount of time.

Don't let the baby use you as a pacifier if your breasts are tender. Each breast is usually emptied during the first ten minutes of nursing (three minutes for the let-down and seven minutes to get the milk out of the breast). After that, although your baby may be getting some milk, he is mainly satisfying his oral needs. If you have sore nipples, try using a pacifier temporarily (preferably a NukSauger) to satisfy his sucking needs. Usually fifteen to twenty minutes on each breast is sufficient to fulfill your baby's needs for nourishment and oral satisfaction.

Be sure your baby has grasped the dark area surrounding the sinus, not just the end of the nipple. If your baby grasps only the end of the nipple, the milk sinus does not reach into his mouth, he cannot squeeze the milk out of the sinus, and the nipple becomes sore. The baby is left hungry and frustrated and the mother upset and anxious.

Remove the baby from your breast properly. Don't pull your baby off your breast while he is sucking. Insert your little finger into his mouth, between the nipple and his lips.

Many women who have successfully established a pattern of scheduled feedings with their babies are horrified to find that suddenly, somewhere around six weeks, their babies are acting like they are starving. The first thought that comes to a new mother's mind is "I've lost my milk!" or "My milk isn't rich enough." But the usual cause is that the baby's appetite has increased in proportion to his growth. When your baby is demanding more, supply more. There is usually a forty-eight-hour period between the balancing of a baby's demand and the mother's capacity to build up the supply he needs. Feeding him more often for longer periods of time quickly builds up your milk supply, and with patience you can once again sit back and relax with a contented baby.

Chapter 8—Problems You May Encounter

Poor Let-Down
Sore Nipples
Engorgement
Lack of Milk Supply

Many of the common problems a new mother may encounter are preventable. However, if a problem does arise and she is not able to overcome it at the onset, it may seriously hamper her success in breast feeding.

During the hospital stay and early days at home you may encounter several situations that can make or break your commitment to breast-feed. Of course, prevention is preferable. But you should be prepared and knowledgeable, for early diagnosis and treatment are of utmost importance in any problem.

POOR LET-DOWN

Cause. Probably the most common cause of failure in breast feeding is the inability to establish a good let-down response. Because let-down is a mental as well as a physical response the best preventative of poor let-down is that a woman be knowledgeable about the process and approach each breast-feeding session relaxed, rested, and with a positive attitude.

Signs. The first indication of poor let-down is that your baby is simply not getting enough milk. He may grasp the nipple voraciously, suck for a little while, satisfied at first by the milk that naturally drains into the reservoirs between feedings, and then become frustrated when the let-down does not take place. The usual signals of let-down, a tingling sensation, fullness of the breast, milk spurting from one or both breasts, uterine contractions, and a slight tenderness in the nipples are not present.

Suggestions. 1. Take positive steps to set up a relaxed and positive atmosphere before feedings.

2. Think positively and surround yourself with support that will boost your confidence.

3. Try to drink a cup of tea or a glass of wine or beer before you start feeding.

4. Before the feeding, apply heat directly to the breasts. Take a hot bath or shower, or use a warm towel or heating pad.

5. After applying heat, gently massage each breast, starting at the base of the breast. While feeding the baby on one side, gently massage the other breast to stimulate let-down.

6. If these steps do not help with let-down, contact your doctor; he can prescribe medication (nasal oxytocin) to enhance your let-down.

Because the let-down is a reflex function, you can help develop it by trying to nurse your baby on a fairly consistent schedule. Continue feeding your baby when he's hungry but begin to try for a three-hour schedule in which you nurse your baby every three hours—even if you have to wake him. Nurse him during the interval if he needs you, but consider this an additional nursing and try again when the three-hour interval comes around.

SORE NIPPLES

Cause. Probably the most common reason women give up nursing their babies in the early stages is sore nipples. A certain amount of tenderness is normal and goes away when your baby continues to nurse. However, sometimes a woman's nipples may continue to hurt. Sore nipples are caused by unprepared and tender nipples being exposed to the prolonged sucking of a nursing baby, and disappear once the nipples have become accustomed to breast feeding.

Signs. A constant tenderness of the nipple area, even when you're not actually nursing, is the first indication. If the condition is allowed to continue, the tenderness may turn to severe pain and the nipples may become cracked. If the nipples aren't treated, they may begin to bleed.

Suggestions. Since sore nipples can lead to infected breasts, it is extremely important that you begin treatment immediately.

1. Call your doctor and follow his advice.

2. Expose nipples to the air and especially to sunshine after each nursing, then rub in Massé, AandD cream, or hydrous lanolin to keep the nipples supple. Rub in the ointment thoroughly so that the nipples can be lubricated but also be exposed to the air.

3. Ask the nurse for a special heat lamp to heal nipples, or use a plain lamp (25 to 50 watts) at home. Some women find that a hair dryer turned directly on the nipples helps to promote healing.

4. Before you begin to nurse, follow steps taken in the let-down treatment (see Index) to enhance let-down.

5. The baby must be allowed to continue nursing. If you stop nursing, the milk ducts may become clogged, which can lead to engorgement and infection.

6. Nurse frequently for short periods.

7. Nurse on the less sore nipple first to enhance let-down, then switch to the other nipple and nurse for a sufficient time to ensure milk drainage. Put your baby on the less sore side to fulfill sucking needs.

8. Nurse frequently to relieve tension on your nipples.

9. Change your baby's sucking position to relieve pain. Many babies have a favorite "side and position," which can exert painful pressure on tender nipples. While nursing, hold the baby's head in your hand rather than with your arm. Or try to hold the "football position" with his head in the hand of the arm on the same side on which you are nursing, hold his body between your side and arm, and let his feet hang out behind.

10. Since sore nipples look and act like a first-degree burn, some women find that crushed ice wrapped in a washcloth and applied *only* to the nipple area between nursings may help relieve and heal sore nipples. Remember, nipple soreness is only temporary and will pass if corrective measures are taken.

ENGORGEMENT

Engorgement is the bugaboo of every nursing mother. If for any reason the milk ducts are not drained completely, there is the possibility that the milk left in the ducts can cause them to become clogged up, and milk from the glands cannot pass through them. The milk glands continue to make milk, the let-down continues to squeeze the milk into the ducts, and the milk tension mounts up, resulting in swelling and tenderness. If the milk is allowed to stagnate in the milk glands they can become infected and extremely painful.

Signs. A woman is usually first aware of engorgement when her breasts become hard, full, and tender. The stretching causes the skin covering the breasts to become shiny and streaked. Because the breasts are swollen, it is difficult for the baby to get the entire dark area into his mouth and he will only get the end of the nipple, causing sore nipples and a hungry and frustrated baby.

Suggestions. It is extremely important that engorgement is treated immediately, to catch it before it turns into mastitis (or infected breasts).
1. Call your doctor immediately, follow his advice, and take any medication he prescribes.
2. Go to bed and take care of yourself.
3. Put ice bags or cold cloths on your breasts between feedings to decrease the swelling and relieve the pain.
4. Right before feeding your baby, put heat on your breasts to enhance the let-down. Fill your tub full of warm water and get in on your hands and knees so your breasts are soaking in the water, or take a warm shower with the water spraying on your breasts. If this isn't possible, get a cloth that has been soaked in hot water and lay it on your breasts.
5. Massage the milk down to the sinus and gently hand-express it out to relieve the fullness and soften the nipple so it is easier for the baby to get hold of. Rough handling can cause more harm than good. Be careful with hot water bottles; the weight of the bottle may be detrimental to the swollen tissue.
6. If only one breast is infected, nurse the baby first on the engorged breast so that it gets the most efficient sucking.
7. Nurse frequently and at short intervals.
8. Rest and take special care of yourself until the swelling, heat, and tenderness subside and your breast feels normal.
9. Hand-express the milk to reduce swelling.
10. Continue to breast-feed at frequent intervals to clear the milk ducts.

LACK OF MILK SUPPLY

Since the amount of milk a mother can produce is determined by how much is sucked out, the more the breasts are emptied the more milk they can produce. It is not uncommon for a new mother to be concerned about how much milk she is capable of producing for her baby. If a baby is not placed on a frequent and flexible schedule to establish a good milk supply, a mother may be concerned that she does not have enough milk. Minimum demand produces a minimum milk supply; maximum demand produces a plentiful milk supply. A poor milk supply can be the by-product of poor let-down and poor drainage.

Signs. Your baby may be cranky and fussy and may act as if he is famished. Because he's not getting enough liquids he is not producing at least six wet diapers a day. The most positive sign is that your baby is losing weight after his normal 10 per cent weight loss at birth.

Suggestions. 1. If you want to build your milk supply, first increase your intake of fluids and ensure that you have an adequate diet with plenty of calcium and protein.
2. Your milk supply is ultimately determined by how much milk your baby consumes, so take positive steps to ensure your let-down function and maintain drainage.
3. Nurse your baby more frequently to build up your supply.
4. If your newborn is losing weight above and beyond his normal weight loss right after birth, be sure to contact your doctor; your baby's welfare is your first concern—not how you feed him.

Chapter 9—Problems a Baby May Encounter

Proper Nursing Position
Crying Baby
Sleepy Baby
Vigorous Nurser
Weak Nurser
Colicky Baby

For breast feeding to succeed, not only is a willing and able mother needed but a willing and able baby as well. And, as nursing is a process of learning for some mothers, so some babies need a little prompting. Just as mothers differ in their ability to breast-feed, so do babies differ in their ability to nurse. Some babies seem to know exactly what to do from minute one; others need instruction. Some of the problems a mother may encounter are a sleepy baby, a crying baby, a weak nurser, a voracious nurser. Each needs special handling. It takes two to tango. A mother may have a tremendous supply of milk to give her baby, and she may have already achieved a good let-down response, but if her baby is unable or unwilling to nurse, he won't get much nourishment. Let's consider some of the problems you may encounter and what you can do about them.

PROPER NURSING POSITION

The first important fact to remember with any baby is that the baby must get its milk from the dark nipple area which covers the reservoirs. Since the size of the areolar region varies in different women, not every woman needs to put the whole areolus into the baby's mouth. The important thing to remember is that your baby must not just grasp the end of the nipple area, but must take in the area with the sinus underneath. If he grasps only the end of the nipple, you are likely to have not only a frustrated and hungry baby, but also a sore nipple.

Correct Position. As your baby begins to nurse, he pulls the whole nipple area into his mouth with a sucking motion. The milk sinuses are now positioned between his tongue and the roof of his mouth. With a

**Sucking
Position**

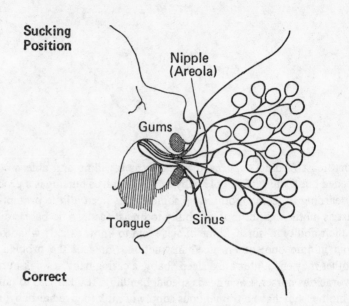

Nipple
(Areola)

Gums

Tongue

Sinus

Correct

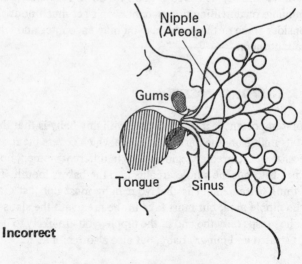

Nipple
(Areola)

Gums

Tongue

Sinus

Incorrect

FIG. 5 SUCKING POSITION

sucking motion he then compresses his gums around the milk sinuses and gently squeezes the milk into his mouth. When the milk gathers in his throat, his swallowing reflex causes him to swallow the milk. When he is nursing properly the long, slow, rhythmical sound of his nursing and his obvious relaxed contentment tell you all is going well.

Incorrect Position. If the baby grasps only the end of the nipple, the milk sinus does not reach into his mouth, and he cannot get the milk out of the sinus. The nipple becomes sore and the baby is left hungry and frustrated. If your baby does not position the nipple between his tongue and palate, he cannot get to the milk sinus to squeeze out its contents. Short, clicky sounds and a squirming, frustrated baby tell you he is not getting at the milk.

CRYING BABY

New babies cry for various reasons. They may be hungry, tired, wet, overstimulated, understimulated, lonely, bored, or in real pain. Crying is their main method of communication. All mothers know the frustration of trying to feed a crying baby. If your baby is crying while you try to feed him, he is liable to become more frustrated and hard to handle. If he is extremely upset, he won't even recognize your breast as a source of nourishment, but as a suffocating obstacle. He'll scream and fight hard to get away from it because he sees it as a threat to his survival. When this happens, don't try to feed him until you can calm him down. It is important to remember that a crying baby is not necessarily a hungry baby.

Suggestions. If it is mealtime, of course, feeding a crying baby is the easiest way to comfort him. If you have already fed him and know he is not hungry, look for other ways to comfort him. Make sure the pins in his diaper are closed. Change his diaper; he may not like to be wet. Try to burp him in case he has an uncomfortable air bubble. Swaddle him snuggly in a warm blanket. Rub his back and tummy; he may have a pain. Put him over your shoulder and walk with him. Sit in a rocking chair and rock him. Croon and talk to him. Put him in a front sling, back-pack, or stroller and take him outside for a walk. Put him in the car and go for a ride. Check to see that he is warm enough, but that he's not too hot. He may simply be bored and wants some attention—

play with him. However, don't overtire or overstimulate him; he needs his sleep too and may be very cranky without it. Your baby is an experienced aquanaut, and he loves the sound and feel of water. Give him a warm bath or run a bath for both of you and let him enjoy the warm water and the feel of being with you. Fill a hot water bottle with warm water or place a hot pad on your lap with your baby on top of it and gently rock him. Put him in the cradle and rock him. Ask all your friends who are experienced mothers what to do. If nothing works, get away from the situation to regain your perspective. Leave him with your husband and go for a walk. Don't be guilty. "God give me the strength to change what I can change, the grace to accept what I can't change, and the wisdom to know the difference." Remember, this situation is temporary.

SLEEPY BABY

New babies can be sleepy babies, especially after an anesthetized delivery. And sleepy babies nurse poorly. A nipple stuffed into an unco-operating mouth is not too well received. Again, don't try to nurse him until you attempt to wake him.

Suggestions. Change his diapers and move him around. Uncover him and expose him to the air; sometimes the change in temperature will shock him awake. Rub his tummy and pat his feet. Talk and play with him. Take him for a brisk walk. Persist in your efforts. Try again in an hour if he doesn't wake up enough to nurse, and every half hour after that. If your baby does not gain the weight he normally should, be sure to contact your doctor. A mother may need to schedule frequent feedings with a sleepy baby for a few weeks so that he nurses enough.

VIGOROUS NURSER

Some babies are overco-operative. This voracious baby gulps his food so vigorously that he tends to take in vast amounts of air that may turn into painful air bubbles later. His vigorous nursing actions can cause extremely painful nipples for his mother. This little tiger needs some prompting and re-education.

Suggestions. Burp your baby before you feed him. Instead of letting him latch onto your nipple with all his vigor, assuage his hunger by massaging your breast and hand-expressing some milk into his mouth. This makes the nipple easier to grasp and calms him down before he starts. When he begins to nurse at the nipple, take him off the breast several times and burp him. When you do take him off the breast, remember not to pull him off, but to break the suction by putting your little finger in between his gums. Don't let your baby nurse too long, because overeating may tend to give him gas bubbles. Use a pacifier temporarily to satisfy his sucking needs. Nurse less frequently; because this baby is such an efficient nurser, he can overeat and get extra gas. If your baby's sucking action causes sore nipples, instead of holding him in the classical arm position, try the "football position." To relieve the pressure on your nipple, hold his head in the hand of the side you are nursing, cradle his body in the crook of your arm like a football, and let his legs dangle behind you.

WEAK NURSER

Some babies, especially premature ones, simply do not have the necessary strength in their mouth muscles to suck milk from their mother's breasts. Babies delivered by Caesarean section or in heavily anesthetized births may not have the strength to nurse well in the beginning. It may be difficult for a baby to empty the breast to establish an adequate milk supply. It is essential that a premature baby get sufficient nourishment, so work closely with your doctor. Your baby's welfare is of primary concern. The weak nurser takes a great deal of patience and time to mature. Remember, this problem is temporary and will fade with time.

Suggestions. Because establishing your milk supply and maintaining drainage is of utmost importance, it is necessary to nurse this type of baby frequently for longer periods of time. Before you begin nursing, massage your breasts and hand-express milk into the baby's mouth to get him to begin nursing. Nurse as long as your baby wants to suck. If the baby cannot empty the breasts, hand massage and express milk to keep the milk ducts from clogging. Keep in close contact with your doctor about your baby's weight gain.

COLICKY BABY

IMMATURE DIGESTIVE SYSTEM.

Some babies are colicky; they cry constantly and seem continually frustrated and uncomfortable even after they are fed, changed and warm, and nothing you do seems to console them. Unfortunately, a mother with a colicky baby is prone to blaming herself. She feels she is doing something wrong and quickly loses confidence in her ability to provide milk for her baby. There are many theories on colic, but little research. However, some doctors feel that colic can be caused by an incompletely developed and immature digestive or nervous system. The baby hasn't developed enough to efficiently ingest and digest his food. It may help to know that colic usually passes by the time a baby is three months old, and some research indicates that babies who are colicky tend to have high intelligence as adults.

OVERACTIVE LET-DOWN.

Colic can also be caused by an overactive let-down system and milk supply. In the early stages of milk production, sometimes the let-down reflex comes with such force that the milk is shot into the baby's mouth, causing him to gulp air in with the milk. Before the colicky baby begins to nurse let the milk spurt out into a jar or bottle until the flow begins to diminish. This situation clears up once your supply becomes balanced to your baby's demands.

Suggestions. Frequent, short feedings seem to be more easily digested by a colicky baby. During the feeding sessions, remove the baby from the breast several times to try to bring up any air bubbles which may have developed. Give your baby lots of love and attention. Be understanding and yet realistic. If the cause seems to be out of your control, don't feel guilty. Anyone loses perspective by being too close to the situation. Get out by yourself and with your husband.

Chapter 10—Change and Challenge

With a new baby, a woman's life changes overnight. Her independent and unconfined life vanishes, and the new mother finds herself with the twenty-four-hour-a-day responsibility of a new human being. Because of the emotional aspects of breast feeding, a new mother who chooses to nurse her baby may be especially affected by these changes. The following section was developed by twenty mothers who attended a seminar on "New Motherhood." They met for over a period of six months, sharing their feelings, concerns, and needs as new mothers. The predominant theme of these meetings was that new mothers felt that they entered motherhood completely unprepared for both the physical and emotional changes which took place in their lives after the birth of their babies. From this seminar came their desire to share their experiences with other new mothers in hope that it would help them view their feelings and concerns as normal. These women developed a series of suggestions which helped them cope with their feelings during the difficult first few weeks. Although these are only the experiences of individual members, we hope to present a spectrum of alternatives from which a new mother can choose, taking what she needs and discarding the rest.

THE MOTHER—WOMAN AND WIFE

New mothers are besieged with feelings ranging from ecstasy to depression. Most women are ashamed to admit feelings of fright, depression, resentment, and inadequacy. After they start talking to each other, they are immensely relieved to discover that their feelings are normal. As their babies mature, they are relieved to find that these feelings are temporary and pass in the first few months.

Many real concerns crop up in the first few weeks. "Will I be a good mother? Will my baby live? Can I cope with the work? Am I giving my husband enough attention? Will I always look so haggard? Do I have enough milk?"

Every new mother needs special protection, love, attention, and ego building. Your husband, family, friends, and doctor (carefully chosen) are all sources of support and confidence.

The difference between realistic and unrealistic expectations of yourself as a mother can mean the difference in your feelings of success or failure. How do you see yourself as a mother? What do you expect of yourself as a wife? What do you want for yourself as a person? Are your expectations realistic?

THE GAMUT OF FEELINGS

Fluctuations of feelings and emotions are normal with the tremendous changes a new baby brings to the family. It is natural for new mothers to have feelings running the gamut from extreme happiness to extreme depression.

FEELINGS OF JOY.

The birth of a baby brings to a woman's life unknown depths of joy, awareness of life, and appreciation.

"I have changed from a partial person to a whole person."

"I am enjoying myself to the fullest and have found a new way of life."

"I find myself growing and changing every day along with my baby."

"I feel myself more whole as a person."

"It's a joy to be part of the creation of a new human being."

"I feel as if I have created a miracle."

"I listen to my baby's heartbeat and am overwhelmed by the significance of this human being who is the total creation of myself and my husband."

"I appreciate my husband and his responsibility to us as a provider."

"I now realize what my parents did and appreciate them more."

"I appreciate the total cycle of life and death."

"I appreciate my own role as a creator."

"I feel proud of my accomplishments."

From the highest feelings of elation with the creation of a new being many new mothers come down to the realism of their twenty-four-hour responsibility. Whereas our grandmothers had the support not only of their own families but of the community they have grown up in, many women in a modern mobile society often find themselves alone in their role as a mother.

PHYSICAL EXHAUSTION.

"I am disappointed. I had great images of myself as a wonderful mother, wife, and person. I am overwhelmed by the amount of work I have. I can't seem to get past the mounds of work piling up. My house is a mess. I can't even seem to get dinner ready on time."

Washing, ironing, cleaning, dusting, changing, feeding, bathing, etc., etc.,—down, down, down from cloud nine. Your miraculous creation with his perfectly shaped nose, mouth, and ears has brought with him a parcel of work and responsibility. Not only that, you have just emerged from the rigorous experience of childbirth. Be realistic; having a baby is hard work. Be prepared for a recuperation period when you come home from the hospital. Some women still experience physical discomfort from their stitches and are coping with a heavy vaginal flow. Your milk may just have come in and you are suffering from engorgement and sore nipples. It is not uncommon for some women to experience the postnatal blues when they first come home from the hospital. Many women feel a letdown much like the day after Christmas. It takes time to adjust to your new role as a mother. Many women are disappointed that they are not the "super-mother" they thought they would be. The unrealistic image of themselves as perfectly made-up, stylishly dressed, calm, patient, understanding, and compassionate is soon dispelled after staying up all night with a crying baby.

Be realistic about your physical resources. If you overtax them during this period, it may take you twice as long to recover and feel like your former self. Don't feel guilty if you don't feel like returning to your active role in the community for the first few months.

Have help in for housework. Don't hesitate to turn to *any* source for help during these first few weeks. Mothers, sisters, friends, and your husband are all sources of relief. A word of caution, however: Surround yourself only with people who are calm, dependable, undemanding, and supportive of breast feeding. If you find your mother, relatives, or friends cannot give you support, their presence may have a negative rather than a positive effect.

Take advantage of the multitude of appliances and services available to you. Diaper service can be surprisingly inexpensive. Disposable diapers for the first few weeks can be a lifesafer. Many public health departments have provisions where a visiting nurse can visit you at no charge. Hired help and a baby sitter during the first few days are far less expensive than the exacting price of emotional and physical depression. You need them for only a short time and the expense is negligible compared to the relief you can get.

Be sure you have plenty of rest. Exhaustion can cut down your milk supply. Don't try to do everything. Let unnecessary chores go. Organize your life so that the important tasks are covered. Those that you leave undone will be there waiting when you get to them.

Don't entertain unless you really want to. Guests mean cleaning, refreshments, dressing up, and entertaining. Many doctors prescribe "no visitors for two weeks," more for the mother than for the baby. Don't entertain people you have to fuss over. If you do want to entertain, invite only those friends you feel comfortable with and who can bring their own refreshments.

Know your limits and don't push too hard. Turn to your husband and share tasks with him. Don't hamper his involvement with the baby by criticizing the way he holds, changes, or bathes the baby. If night feedings are exhausting you, have your husband bring the baby to you and stay in bed to nurse, napping while you are feeding him.

TENSION AND FATIGUE.

"I am constantly tired and tense. I can't seem to get enough sleep. I'm overwhelmed. I feel my work is never done; it piles up far faster than I can accomplish it. My house is a mess. Dinner is never ready on time. I look like a haggard housewife. I resent the fact that I don't have any time to myself."

Every new mother (and father) is unprepared for the reduced hours of sleep she gets for the first six weeks. Her baby never knew a clock schedule when he was in her uterus, and he's not about to accept such limits during the first few weeks. Unrealistic expectations sometimes make it very hard for a young mother to accustom herself to the constant needs of a newborn. She is not only awake to give him feedings every two or three hours, but she may also lie awake listening for her baby, and sometimes she has a hard time going back to sleep after the night feedings. Not only is our new mother tired from lack of sleep, but she is also overwhelmed by the amount of work her new creation has brought into her life. An experienced mother knows there are many ways she can cut down on the demands of her new baby. She has realistic expectations of her baby's needs and is realistic about her own resources of energy.

Tension is the great exhauster. When you are tense it is hard to organize your thoughts and actions. Define and analyze your patterns of tension. Are you most tense in the morning, staring at the piles of work to be done, is it right before your husband comes home, or is it during night feedings?

Be sure to get enough rest. Forget the piles of work and nap while your baby is napping. Nurse your baby while lying down. Your letdown is enhanced when you are relaxed and rested. A hot bath or shower will help you relax and sleep.

The responsibilities of a new baby are sometimes so demanding that you may forget to get adequate exercise. Exercise makes your body feel better and react more efficiently. Get out for a brisk walk at least once a day. Fresh air and sunshine will help revitalize your spirits and give you a fresh perspective of your life.

There are many good books on relaxation techniques. Read these and find your own special pattern of relaxation. Take time to listen to good music and save a special book and use it as your own special time to relax and temporarily forget all the demands on you. Avoid distressful situations or people who make you tense.

Nap once or twice a day (take the phone off the hook) without feeling guilty.

LACK OF CONFIDENCE.

"I am bewildered by the overwhelming responsibility of my new baby. I hardly know where to begin or who to turn to."

Most women experience a feeling of tremendous responsibility with their unfamiliar role as a mother. They lack not only knowledge but also someone to give them confidence and support. They suffer not only from ignorance, but also from unrealistic expectations for themselves and their new babies.

During these early days, a new mother judges herself on how well she is able to comfort her child. Some lucky mothers have babies who are a sheer delight. That is, they cry very little and sleep a lot. These women may congratulate themselves on what good mothers they are. Other women may have babies who cry a lot and sleep very little. Although this period may only last a few weeks, to the mother it seems to last an eternity. If a mother can't comfort her baby she begins to lack confidence in herself as a mother, person, and wife. Mothers with many children realize that right from birth babies have their own definite personalities. One baby may be "perfect" (i.e. he doesn't cry) and another may be inconsolable. If you have a fussy baby, you will be able to cope better with the situation if you can view it with some perspective.

Don't blame yourself for a fussy baby. Instead of feeling guilty, remember that your baby is making a lot of physical adjustments these first few weeks. Do what you can to comfort him (see Appendix under Crying Baby), and then accept the situation realistically. If your baby is fussy, comfort him and then go out for a walk by yourself, if possible. If you remain too close to the situation, your perspective becomes distorted and it is difficult to remain realistic.

Be yourself. Don't try to be a "super-mother." Don't try to impress others. Be confident that you have natural instincts to do the right thing at the right time. If you feel strongly that you cannot leave your baby to cry, don't. Pick him up and cuddle him. On the other hand, if you feel you have done all you can, don't be worried about letting him cry. Experienced mothers seem to have a sixth sense about the important cries and those they can do nothing about.

Contrary to all the literature you read in women's magazines (run by men editors), you are not going to ruin your baby. Kids are resilient and can cope with more than we give them credit for; the whole history of mankind bears this out.

Pick a doctor in whom you have confidence and who respects you as an individual and gives you confidence in yourself. You *do* know your baby better than anyone else does. You *do* know when things are going right. And you *do* know when things are going wrong. Find a doctor you feel comfortable with, whom you respect and whom you can count on. Don't feel guilty about changing doctors. All doctors are human and realize that there can be a personality clash between them and their patients.

Count on your husband as a friend and confidant. Tell him how you feel—he may be feeling the same way. Give each other mutual support. Lean on friends who have been through the same experience and can give you help, sympathy, and support.

There are voluminous amounts of literature on the care of new babies. Visit your library and bookstore and load up on the information; making use of the information you feel comfortable with and which fits your style, and discarding the rest.

There are many groups of new mothers who lend invaluable support to you. Look in the telephone book for a La Leche group which can give you excellent support. Search out groups sponsored by the Red Cross and YWCA, or call your local hospital for other groups in your community.

Involve your husband. It is always amazing how well a husband can figure out a problem which may be overwhelming to you, who are so close to the baby. Your husband can logically analyze and figure out a solution. Remember, it's his baby too.

CONFINEMENT.

"I was always free, but I didn't appreciate it. I think I resent the lack of freedom now more than anything else. I sometimes feel like I'm a prisoner in my own home. Taking a walk by myself is a major victory. I'm so confined that I feel I can't see the forest for the trees."

Because a new baby has many real needs that must be met, it is not unnatural for a woman to have feelings of being confined. Although this period passes as the baby matures, a new mother can easily become overwhelmed by the situation. Take special care that you don't feel imprisoned by your baby.

New babies travel well. Put your baby in a front-pack or other carrier at least once a day and get out for a walk. Babies are hardy beings and can go almost anywhere. They thrive on action, noise, and activity. Don't turn down a chance to go to a movie or restaurant. Bundle up your baby and take him right along. Hiking and camping are wonderful sports for you, your husband, and your baby. Back-pack carriers can change your life—get one. Husbands seem much more willing to assume baby responsibilities with a back-pack carrier.

Hire a baby sitter you feel confident about and go out with your husband, get out with friends and go out shopping by yourself. Some women hire a baby sitter to take care of the baby while they stay at home to read, sleep, take a bath, or do something they enjoy in private.

Don't feel guilty about leaving your baby with your husband. This gives them time together without mother hovering between them.

Don't bury your guilt feelings. Seek support from a group and from friends who will share their feelings with you. You will be relieved to find that these feelings are normal and you don't have to feel guilty about normal feelings.

A new baby will stress the free time your husband and you had before its arrival. You both must be realistic and mature in realizing that a newborn has real needs; aware that this time will pass, and mindful of the importance of working at your marriage.

GUILT.

"I feel guilty if I leave my baby crying, and then I feel guilty if I pick him up all the time. I also feel that I am not giving my husband all the time he deserves."

Lack of knowledge and confidence in your role as a mother can sometimes contribute to feelings of doubt and guilt. One magazine article says to do one thing and another authority tells you to do another. Many women just don't know what is the right thing to do and are left with nagging feelings of guilt.

Have faith in your own instincts about what is right. If your baby is crying and you want to pick him up, pick him up. If your baby has been crying all day and you know he has been fed, changed, and cared for and you don't feel like picking him up for the moment, don't pick him up.

You are not superhuman. Decide priorities for both your needs and your baby's needs—realizing that certain needs have to be met first. It's healthy to think about yourself and your needs and it's okay to want to do things that don't involve your baby.

CHANGING FAMILY SCENE

RELATIONSHIP WITH YOUR HUSBAND.

"I feel that my relationship with my husband is closer and more profound than it ever has been. I worry, however, that we don't have enough time together to share our feelings."

The coming of a new baby brings many changes. Your role has changed from wife and person to wife, mother, and person. Your baby is not just an eight-hour-a-day job, but a twenty-four-hour responsibility. The first few weeks of a baby's life revolve around his mother. Many women are naturally anxious about the effect of this on their relationship with their husbands.

Put yourself in your husband's shoes. How would you feel if you had been living with a person who was free to give all of the love and attention to you, night and day. The house was in order and meals were on time. Suddenly a new person comes into the household and life changes radically. Colic, rashes, diarrhea, and spit-ups become familiar occurrences. The house is a mess and there are diapers in the toilet. Dinner is never ready on time. And on top of it all, that love and energy that used to be given to the husband is being directed to the baby.

It is a wise wife who understands the special needs of her husband during this period. The father of a newborn undergoes traumatic changes in his feelings about himself, his wife, and his baby. A man has concerns about his ability to assume his role as a father and provider. A man needs special attention, tenderness, and understanding at this stage. He must not only be needed, but appreciated as well.

Fatherhood is not spontaneous. Don't be disillusioned if it takes a while for your husband to become accustomed to his role as a father. Share feelings with each other, and remember that both high and low feelings are common at this state. Your dependence and need for support from your husband are greater than ever. However, don't be unrealistic in your expectations from your husband. His needs for support are probably as great as yours. Above all, remember that this stage is temporary—it won't go on forever.

Special efforts at pleasing your husband will be well received. Dress up for him, prepare a dinner with candlelight and a glass of wine. Get a baby sitter and go out together at least once a week to get a perspective on your relationship. Tell him you appreciate him and thank him for his help. Try to keep in touch with where he is, how he feels, and what upsets him.

SEXUAL ADJUSTMENTS.

Recent research from SEICUS has brought out the need for sexual intercourse in a couple's life after childbirth. After a baby is born into a family, the husband is especially needful of affection, attention, and love. A woman needs the security, protection, and love that sex can signify. A couple re-establishes their relationship in sexual intercourse. With a new baby around, it is sometimes the only time they can be alone to reaffirm their love for one another.

Clinical research has shown that a woman may resume sexual intercourse whenever she is physically and emotionally ready for it. There is no reason to prohibit intercourse after childbirth once the vaginal bleeding has stopped and any incision in the vaginal outlet has healed. However, many new mothers are concerned with the changes that take place in their sex lives and the adjustments which have to be made.

Very few mothers are at all prepared for the twenty-four-hour schedule of a new baby and all the accompanying work. When—or if—they do make it to bed with their husbands, they feel too fatigued to engage in the playfulness of pre-baby days.

A new mother feels that her first responsibility is to her baby. If the baby begins to cry while a couple is attempting intercourse, the mother is usually turned off immediately, because her enjoyment of sex is mental as well as physical.

It is not uncommon for a new mother to be flowing heavily and experiencing discomfort from the stitches of childbirth. Her breasts may be engorged and the nipples sore. Under these circumstances, sexual intercourse is probably the last thing she is interested in. However, the act of sexual intercourse is not the only way to show love to one another. Touching, cuddling, and massage are all essential parts of meaningful lovemaking.

Some of the women mentioned that they were unpleasantly surprised that a previously healthy sex drive was diminished after childbirth. Without lubrication, intercourse can be painful and unpleasant to a woman. After childbirth, the vaginal area may lack lubrication, and this makes intercourse uncomfortable. During breast feeding the secretion of hormones may cause lack of vaginal moisture. Many women find that although they had never used artificial lubrication before childbirth, the use of it during at least the first few occasions of intercourse makes a great deal of difference.

If a woman is responding to her husband, she may experience involuntary leaking of her breasts during intercourse. Some women expressed feelings of guilt and embarrassment at this phenomenon. Others said their husbands found it amusing or even erotic. Don't be concerned, leaking breasts are indicative of a pleasurable response to sex.

Chapter 11–Summary

Keys to Successful Breast Feeding
Problems—Mother
Problems—Baby

KEYS TO SUCCESSFUL BREAST FEEDING

Personal Commitment to Breast Feeding. The first vital ingredient in breast feeding is a woman who really wants to breast-feed.

Support of Husband. Because of the importance of your husband's support, the decision you make should be mutual. A woman who is supported by her husband can almost always have a good experience. Before your husband comes to a decision he also should have some information on the advantages of breast feeding to both you and your baby.

Knowledge. An understanding of milk production, let-down, adequate drainage, and milk supply can prevent many of the problems that lead to failure. Understanding prevention and knowing what to do if problems arise are vital to a good experience.

Preparation. Although not all women need to prepare their breasts, preparation of nipples and breasts help to prevent problems after the baby is born.

Confidence. Confidence in your innate ability to produce milk is a vital ingredient to breast feeding.

Supportive Doctor, Nurse, and Hospital Policy. Choose a doctor who will support you both before and after the birth of your baby. A helpful nurse can give you information and help that will help set you off to a good start. Check into "rooming-in" and "family-centered maternity care" in the hospitals you have in your area.

Early First Nursing Experience. The earlier the first experience, the better for you and your baby. It helps to avoid engorgement and allows for a closeness between you and your baby.

Frequent Nursing on a Flexible Schedule. To avoid engorgement, maintain drainage, and build up a good milk supply, nurse your baby when he's hungry.

Avoid Exhaustion. Rest and relaxation are probably the most important aspects of successful breast feeding. Tension and fatigue can seriously diminish a milk supply. Rest and relaxation can enhance your milk supply. Avoid exhaustion.

Supplements. It's generally agreed that until you feel comfortable about your milk supply it is better to avoid supplements. Because your milk supply is dependent upon how much milk is sucked out by your baby, supplements (that is, formula, water, solids, and even in some cases, pacifiers) can affect your milk.

Helpful Friends. It is extremely helpful to have a friend who has successfully breast-fed her baby and to whom you can turn to for advice and support. If at all possible, contact a breast-feeding group (such as La Leche), who can give you knowledgeable information and support when you need it.

PROBLEMS—MOTHER

LACK OF SUPPLY.

Cause: Principle—Minimum demand produces minimum supply; maximum demand produces plentiful supply. A baby placed on a rigid, infrequent schedule may not be able to empty the breasts and cannot establish a good milk supply. A poor milk supply can also be the by-product of poor drainage and poor let-down reflex.

SIGNS OF A POOR SUPPLY.

1. Inadequate weight gain
2. Fewer than six wet diapers a day
3. Unhappy baby

Demand and Supply

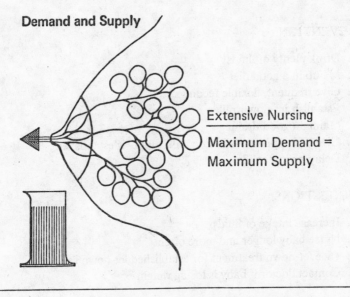

Extensive Nursing

Maximum Demand =
Maximum Supply

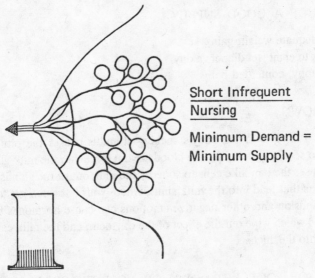

Short Infrequent
Nursing

Minimum Demand =
Minimum Supply

Minimum demand = minimum supply
Maximum demand = maximum supply

FIG. 6 DEMAND AND SUPPLY

PREVENTION.

1. Drink plenty of fluids
2. Maintain a good diet
3. Give frequent, flexible feedings
4. Establish let-down reflex
5. Maintain good drainage
6. Give no supplements before milk supply is established
7. Delay giving solids

SUGGESTIONS.

1. Increase intake of fluids
2. Nurse baby longer and more often
3. (See let-down treatment for established let-down reflex)
4. Contact doctor if baby is losing weight

SIGNS OF A GOOD SUPPLY.

1. Adequate weight gain
2. Six to eight wet diapers a day
3. Happy, contented baby

LET-DOWN.

Cause: Principle—Your baby's sucking stimulus causes the pituitary gland to send oxytocin into the bloodstream; it reaches the milk glands and causes the bandlike cells to squeeze the milk out of the glands into the ducts that lead into the milk sinus, where your baby can get to the milk. Tension and other negative emotions can cause hormones to be secreted which wipe out the effect of the oxytocin, and the milk cannot be let into the ducts.

SIGNS OF POOR LET-DOWN OR NO LET-DOWN.

1. Baby obviously not getting milk, fussy while breast-feeding
2. No milk spurting
3. No sensation of let-down

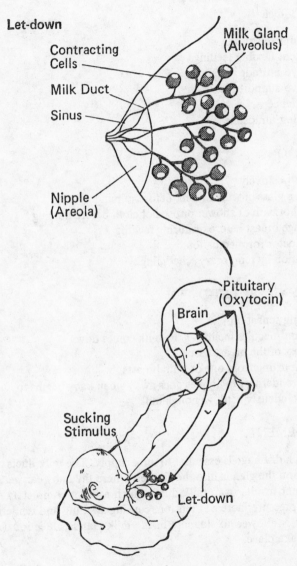

Let-down

Milk Gland (Alveolus)

Contracting Cells

Milk Duct

Sinus

Nipple (Areola)

Pituitary (Oxytocin)

Brain

Sucking Stimulus

Let-down

Baby at breast

FIG. 7 LET-DOWN

PREVENTION.

1. Rest and relaxation
2. Frequent flexible feedings
3. Positive attitude
4. Positive support
5. Confidence
6. Soothing atmosphere

SUGGESTIONS.

1. Think positively
2. Drink a glass of wine or beer before nursing
3. Take hot bath or shower or use hot cloth before nursing
4. Massage breast before or during feeding
5. Call doctor for medication
6. Condition by temporary scheduling

SIGNS OF GOOD LET-DOWN.

1. Tingling sensation
2. Pins-and-needles feeling as the milk comes down
3. Fullness of the breast tissue
4. Milk spurting from one or both breasts
5. Slight tenderness in nipples goes away when baby begins to nurse
6. Baby obviously getting enough milk

ENGORGEMENT.

Cause: Milk drainage is essential to milk supply. The milk ducts carry the milk from the glands into the sinuses, where the baby can get to it. Engorgement results from milk ducts which are not completely emptied. Milk pressure increases tension, causing swelling and tenderness. If the milk is allowed to stagnate in the milk glands, infection (mastitis) can take place.

SIGNS OF ENGORGEMENT.

1. Fullness and hardness in breast tissue
2. Swelling tissue

Maintain Drainage

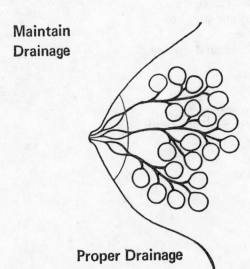

Proper Drainage

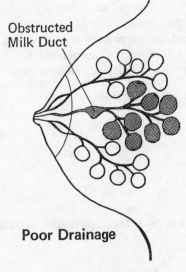

Obstructed Milk Duct

Poor Drainage

FIG. 8 DRAINAGE

3. Lump in the breast (clogged duct)
4. Skin may be shiny and stretched
5. Tenderness
6. Red and hot and painful if infected

PREVENTION.

1. Preparation in pregnancy
2. Nurse as soon as possible after birth
3. Nurse frequently
4. Lots of rest
5. No missed feedings

SUGGESTIONS.

1. Treat immediately
2. Call doctor
3. Go to bed and rest
4. Put ice bags or cold cloths on breasts between feedings to minimize swelling
5. Put hot water on breast before feeding to enhance let-down
6. Put baby on engorged side first
7. Massage breasts and hand-express to reduce swelling
8. Nurse frequently at short intervals to clear ducts
9. Nurse for shorter periods to preclude painfulness

SIGNS OF RECOVERY.

1. Swelling subsides
2. Tenderness and heat subsides
3. Breasts feel normal

SORE NIPPLES.

Cause: Sore nipples are caused by unfamiliar pressure on unprepared, tender nipples.

SIGNS OF SORE NIPPLES.

1. Constant tenderness of the nipple area even after the baby has begun to nurse

**Sucking
Position**

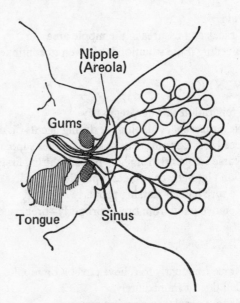

Nipple
(Areola)

Gums

Tongue

Sinus

Correct

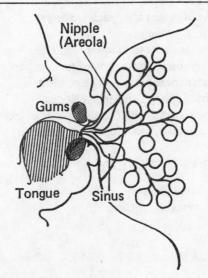

Nipple
(Areola)

Gums

Tongue

Sinus

Incorrect

Proper sucking technique

FIG. 9 SUCKING POSITION

2. Pain
3. Cracks and fissures in the nipple area
4. Bleeding if the situation is allowed to continue

PREVENTION.

1. Preparation during pregnancy
2. Never use soap, alcohol, or drying agents on nipples
3. Use Massé or ointment to keep nipples supple
4. Nurse frequently for short periods during first few days
5. Don't let baby use you as a pacifier
6. Be sure baby is nursing properly
7. Remove baby from breast properly—break suction with finger

SUGGESTIONS.

1. Nurse frequently to relieve tension on nipples
2. Call doctor immediately
3. Expose nipples to air after nursing
4. Use ointment after each feeding
5. Use heat lamp
6. Use let-down techniques before feeding
7. Nurse on less sore nipple first to enhance let-down
8. Nurse for short period on sore side
9. Change baby's sucking positions
10. Use breast shield if unable to nurse directly on nipple
11. Remember, sore nipples are temporary and will pass

SIGNS OF RECOVERY.

1. Less tenderness
2. No cracking or bleeding

PROBLEMS—BABY

SLEEPY BABY.

Cause: New baby
        Anesthetized birth

SUGGESTIONS.

1. Change diapers
2. Move him around, jostle him gently
3. Uncover and expose to air
4. Rub tummy and pat feet
5. Talk and play with him
6. Take for brisk walk
7. Persist every half hour
8. Call doctor for persistent weight loss
9. Situation is temporary
10. Mother may need to schedule baby for a while

TOO VIGOROUS NURSER.

Cause: Overco-operative baby

SUGGESTIONS.

1. Burp baby before you feed him
2. Massage breast and hand-express milk into his mouth
3. Take him off breast several times and burp him
4. Remove baby from breast properly
5. Don't let baby nurse too long
6. Give him a pacifier to satisfy sucking needs

WEAK NURSER.

Cause: Premature baby
        Caesarean section
        Anesthetized delivery
        Immature development of sucking muscles

SUGGESTIONS.

1. Nurse baby frequently for longer periods of time
2. Massage and hand-express milk to begin nursing
3. Nurse as long as baby wants
4. Hand-massage and express milk to maintain drainage

5. Remember, situation is temporary and will pass
6. Keep in contact with doctor if baby does not gain enough weight

CRYING.

Cause: Hunger
       Fatigue
       Loneliness
       Boredom
       Wet diaper
       Pain

SUGGESTIONS.

1. Feed him
2. Check for pin or other physical reasons for discomfort
3. Check for air bubble
4. Swaddle him in warm blanket
5. Rub back and tummy
6. Put over shoulder and walk with him
7. Sit in rocking chair and rock him
8. Croon and talk to him
9. Sing loudly
10. Put in sling, back-pack, or stroller and go out
11. Put in car and go for a ride
12. Make sure he's warm enough
13. Check to see if he's too hot
14. Play with him
15. Let him get his sleep
16. Give him a warm bath
17. Rock him on hot water bottle
18. Put in cradle and rock him
19. Give him a pacifier
20. Ask advice from experienced mother
21. Leave him with your husband
22. Go for a walk by yourself
23. Get a baby sitter and go out with husband
24. Don't feel guilty
25. Situation is temporary

COLICKY BABY.

Theory—immature digestive system (no one really knows).
Immature nervous system

SUGGESTIONS.

1. Frequent, short feeding
2. Frequent burpings
3. Lots of love, body contact, skin caressing
4. Understanding
5. Realism
6. Getting out to gain perspective
7. No guilt

OVERACTIVE LET-DOWN

Remove baby when experiencing let-down to let milk spurt
Before feeding let milk spurt—diminish flow
Hand-express to get rid of excess milk
Soften breasts so baby can get to nipple
Burp baby before feedings
Frequent burping during feedings
Let pacifier satisfy sucking needs

APPENDIX

Listing of contacts for breast-feeding help or information about local meetings:
A.S.P.O. (Association Society for Psychoprophylaxis in Obstetrics)
1523 L Street N.W.
Washington, D.C. 20005

I.C.E.A. (International Childbirth Education Association)
809 Oxford Road
Ann Arbor, Michigan 48104

LA LECHE LEAGUE INTERNATIONAL
9616 Minneapolis Avenue
Franklin Park, Illinois 60131

The following is a listing of the phone numbers for the state offices of La Leche League:

Alabama: see *Georgia*
Alaska: see *Washington*
Arizona: 602-296-1172 or 602-992-5625
Arkansas: see *Louisiana*
California (Northern): 415-325-4337 or 408-262-3571
California (Southern): 213-395-4680 or 213-425-1341
Colorado: 303-771-3554 or 303-428-1009
Connecticut: 203-743-1662 or 203-354-9649
Delaware: see *Maryland*
District of Columbia: see *Maryland*
Florida: 305-752-4873 or 904-744-2361
Georgia: 404-636-9780
Hawaii: 808-677-0461 or 808-689-7402
Idaho: see *Oregon*
Illinois: 312-627-9516 or 213-584-4999
Indiana: 317-291-8847 or 317-293-4417

Iowa: 515-266-9720 or 319-391-5409
Kansas: 316-663-4716 or 913-273-0042
Kentucky: 502-634-0025 or 606-278-8387
Louisiana: 318-235-2809 or 318-757-4856
Maine: 1-207-882-7290
Maryland: 301-652-2314 or 301-577-4210
Massachusetts: 413-596-6657
Michigan: 517-631-4871 or 616-381-7185
Minnesota: 612-483-5679 or 612-756-9300
Mississippi: 601-922-5466
Missouri: 816-781-6622 or 816-763-0188
Montana: 406-656-1495
Nebraska: 402-564-7776 or 308-882-5170
Nevada: see *Southern California*
New Hampshire: 1-603-225-2581 or 1-603-673-4803
New Jersey: 201-584-3187 or 201-463-8363
New Mexico: see *Arizona*
New York: 716-282-0909 or 518-279-3973
North Carolina: 704-366-0712 or 919-489-8085
North Dakota: 701-225-8779
Ohio: 614-268-4685 or 513-325-0044
Oklahoma: 405-364-3814
Oregon: 503-292-0821
Pennsylvania: 814-899-3438
Rhode Island: 401-294-6520
South Carolina: see *North Carolina*
South Dakota: 605-648-3205
Tennessee: 615-889-4755
Texas: 214-339-2908 or 512-836-2518
Utah: 801-262-2230
Vermont: see *Massachusetts*
Virginia: see *Maryland*
Washington: 206-385-1506 or 206-243-2811
West Virginia: see *Maryland*
Wyoming: see *Montana*

Outside of U.S.A.:

Canada: 416-488-3368 or 416-765-2892

Other groups: For further information, 312-832-6790 or 312-532-3201 or 312-231-8155

SUGGESTED READING

Eiger, Marion S., M.D. and Sally Wendkos Olds
The Complete Book of Breastfeeding
New York: The Workman Publishing Company, Inc., 1972.

Gerard, Alice
Please Breast Feed Your Baby
New York: New American Library, 1971.

Jelliffe, D. B. and E. F. Jelliffe
"The Significance of Human Milk" (a symposium)
American Journal of Clinical Nutrition (August 1971)

Niles Newton
The Family Book of Child Care
New York: Harper, 1957.

Pryor, Karen
Nursing Your Baby
New York: Harper & Row, 1963.

La Leche League International
The Womanly Art of Breastfeeding
Franklin Park, Ill.: La Leche League International, 1963.

INDEX

bleeding), 7, 91, 98. *See also* Menstrual cycle

Vigorous nursers, 84–85, 113

Virus, viral infections, 6, 7

Visiting nurses, 92

Vitamin C, 6

Vitamin D, 6

Vitamin E, 6

Vomiting, 6

Walking with babies, 95
 crying, 83

Water, for crying babies, 84

Weak nursers, 18–19, 85, 113–14

Weaning, 63

Weight, 31, 53, 77, 84
 formulas and gain in, 6
 premature babies and, 19
 and weak nursers, 85

Wine, before nursing, 74

Womanly Art of Breastfeeding, The, 118

Woolrich shield, 43

Working, 13–14

YWCA, 95